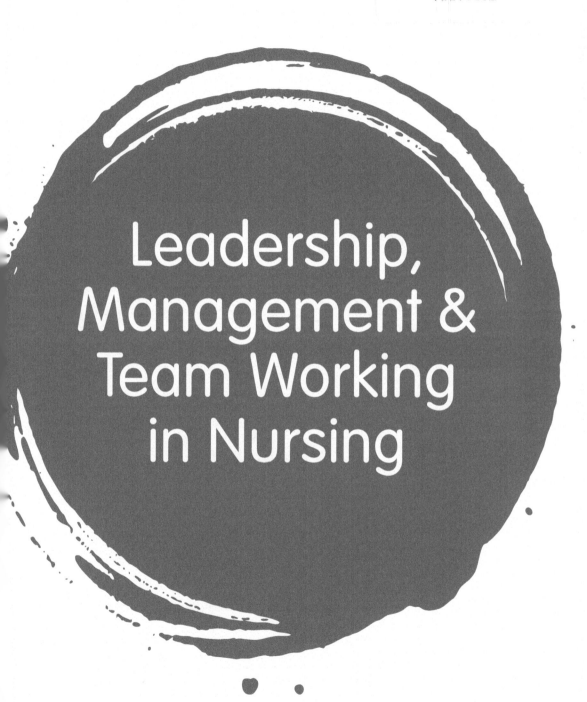

Leadership, Management & Team Working in Nursing

Sara Miller McCune founded SAGE Publishing in 1965 to support the dissemination of usable knowledge and educate a global community. SAGE publishes more than 1000 journals and over 800 new books each year, spanning a wide range of subject areas. Our growing selection of library products includes archives, data, case studies and video. SAGE remains majority owned by our founder and after her lifetime will become owned by a charitable trust that secures the company's continued independence.

Los Angeles | London | New Delhi | Singapore | Washington DC | Melbourne

Leadership, Management & Team Working in Nursing

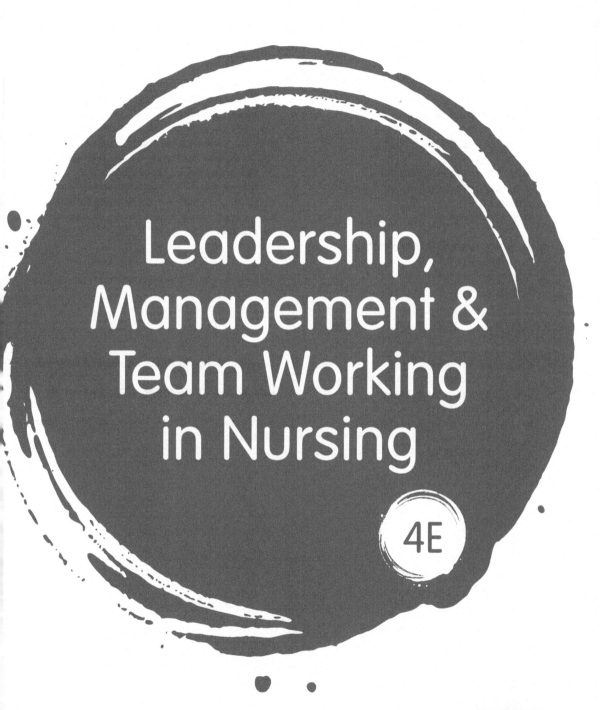

4E

Peter Ellis

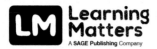

Learning Matters
A SAGE Publishing Company
1 Oliver's Yard
55 City Road
London EC1Y 1SP

SAGE Publications Inc.
2455 Teller Road
Thousand Oaks, California 91320

SAGE Publications India Pvt Ltd
B 1/I 1 Mohan Cooperative Industrial Area
Mathura Road
New Delhi 110 044

SAGE Publications Asia-Pacific Pte Ltd
3 Church Street
#10-04 Samsung Hub
Singapore 049483

Editor: Laura Walmsley
Development editor: Richenda Milton-Daws
Senior project editor: Chris Marke
Project management: River Editorial
Marketing manager: Ruslana Khatagova
Cover design: Sheila Tong
Typeset by: C&M Digitals (P) Ltd, Chennai, India
Printed in the UK

Library of Congress Control Number: 2021944696

British Library Cataloguing in Publication Data

A catalogue record for this book is available from the British Library

ISBN 978-1-5297-7372-9
ISBN 978-1-5297-7371-2 (Pbk)

At SAGE we take sustainability seriously. Most of our products are printed in the UK using responsibly sourced papers and boards. When we print overseas we ensure sustainable papers are used as measured by the PREPS grading system. We undertake an annual audit to monitor our sustainability.

Contents

About the author		viii
Foreword		ix
	Introduction	1
1	Experience of management and leadership	4
2	Frameworks for management and leadership	25
3	Teams and teamwork	49
4	Working with individuals in teams	69
5	Conflict management and negotiation skills	89
6	Coaching, mentoring and clinical supervision	109
7	Improving care and change management	129
8	Creating a learning environment	153
9	Developing confidence as a manager and leader	170
Glossary		188
References		190
Index		200

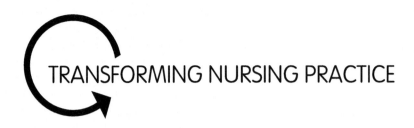

TRANSFORMING NURSING PRACTICE

Transforming Nursing Practice is a series tailor made for pre-registration student nurses. Each book in the series is:

 Affordable

 Full of active learning features

 Mapped to the NMC Standards of proficiency for registered nurses

 Focused on applying theory to practice

Each book addresses a core topic and they have been carefully developed to be simple to use, quick to read and written in clear language.

An invaluable series of books that explicitly relates to the NMC standards. Each book covers a different topic that students need to explore in order to develop into a qualified nurse... I would recommend this series to all Pre-Registered nursing students whatever their field or year of study.

LINDA ROBSON,
Senior Lecturer at Edge Hill University

Many titles in the series are on our recommended reading list and for good reason - the content is up to date and easy to read. These are the books that actually get used beyond training and into your nursing career.

EMMA LYDON,
Adult Student Nursing

ABOUT THE SERIES EDITORS

DR MOOI STANDING is an Independent Nursing Consultant (UK and International) and is responsible for the core knowledge, adult nursing and personal and professional learning skills titles. She is an experienced NMC Quality Assurance Reviewer of educational programmes and Professional Regulator Panellist on the NMC Practice Committee. Mooi is also Board member of Special Olympics Malaysia, enabling people with intellectual disabilities to participate in sports and athletics nationally and internationally.

DR SANDRA WALKER is a Clinical Academic in Mental Health working between Southern Health Trust and the University of Southampton and responsible for the mental health nursing titles. She is a Qualified Mental Health Nurse with a wide range of clinical experience spanning more than 25 years.

BESTSELLING TEXTBOOKS

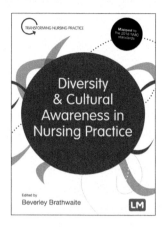

Diversity & Cultural Awareness in Nursing Practice

Edited by Beverley Brathwaite

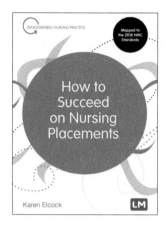

How to Succeed on Nursing Placements

Karen Elcock

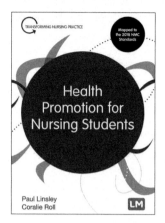

Health Promotion for Nursing Students

Paul Linsley
Coralie Roll

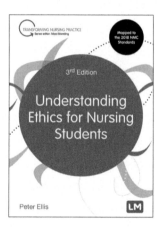

3rd Edition

Understanding Ethics for Nursing Students

Peter Ellis

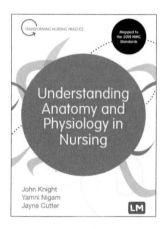

Understanding Anatomy and Physiology in Nursing

John Knight
Yamni Nigam
Jayne Cutter

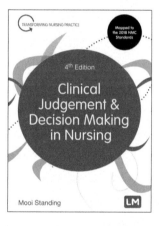

4th Edition

Clinical Judgement & Decision Making in Nursing

Mooi Standing

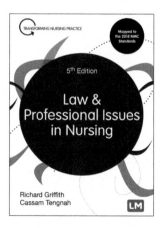

5th Edition

Law & Professional Issues in Nursing

Richard Griffith
Cassam Tengnah

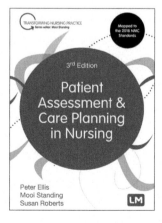

3rd Edition

Patient Assessment & Care Planning in Nursing

Peter Ellis
Mooi Standing
Susan Roberts

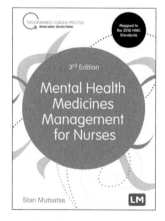

3rd Edition

Mental Health Medicines Management for Nurses

Stan Mutsatsa

You can find a full list of textbooks in the *Transforming Nursing Practice* series at

https://uk.sagepub.com

About the author

Peter Ellis is an independent nursing and health and social care writer and consultant. Peter was most recently a registered manager and nursing director in the hospice and social care settings. Prior to this, he was a senior lecturer and programme director at Canterbury Christ Church University where he taught leadership and management, among other topics, to undergraduate and postgraduate students. Peter is also an Honorary Senior Research Fellow of Canterbury Christ Church University and has a special interest, including ongoing research, in palliative and end-of-life care.

Foreword

Leadership, Management and Team Working in Nursing engages readers in a step-by-step exploration, ranging from reflecting on how they like to be managed, to understanding how they can be more effective team players, co-ordinators and leaders in person-centred care. One of the main strengths of the book is the way in which it succinctly integrates relevant management and leadership theory with nursing values and the practicalities of delivering high standards of care within complex multidisciplinary healthcare organisations. It does so by continually drawing parallels between the qualities of a good nurse and a good leader. For example: being self-aware of one's own development needs; accepting and respecting individual differences and cultural diversity; creating a collaborative, nurturing culture which maximises the contribution and development of all parties; listening to, negotiating with and caring for colleagues as well as patients; developing emotional intelligence and resilience in managing stressful events; and inspiring trust in others through one's competence, values and professional commitment. This is very helpful in enabling readers to integrate their understanding of themselves as individual nurses, as members of a multidisciplinary team and as employees of organisations responsible for providing safe and effective healthcare. As such, it is essential reading for all nursing students so they can understand where they 'fit in' and the important contribution they can make to the healthcare team in delivering care.

Each chapter is mapped against relevant standards of proficiency for nurses (NMC, 2018a); for example, Platform 5 'Leading nursing care and working in teams'. Collectively they inform compliance with *The Code* (NMC, 2018b), such as: *25. Provide leadership to make sure people's wellbeing is protected and to improve their experiences of the healthcare system.* The book is therefore essential reading for nursing students in understanding and developing their skills in leadership, management and team working for the benefit of all service users. I also recommend the book to registered nurses as it will be an invaluable resource when reflecting upon their care management and leadership skills for NMC (Nursing and Midwifery Council) revalidation purposes. The fourth edition has been updated, reflecting feedback from reviewers, new reference sources and the impact of a coronavirus pandemic on nursing leadership and management.

Peter Ellis has skillfully combined his extensive nursing, educational and managerial expertise in an excellent book packed with real-life case studies and stimulating activities, thereby enabling nursing students and registered nurses to apply relevant management theory to enhance their nursing practice. I hope you enjoy reading it as much as I did.

Dr Mooi Standing, Series Editor

Introduction

Leadership is a key feature of twenty-first-century nursing. The interdisciplinary requirements of modern healthcare, the multiplicity of nursing and nursing support roles and increasing demands of an ageing population all mean the co-ordination of care is more complex now than it was at any time in the past.

The need for strong, supportive, interdisciplinary leadership has been widely demonstrated during the COVID-19 pandemic. This unprecedented challenge has caused leaders in health and social care to take stock of the ways in which they work and communicate with their teams. In this edition of the book, we draw on some of the ongoing learning for nurse leadership which has emerged and is emerging from this pandemic.

We also explore many facets of the leadership role and what these mean for nurses. As with training to become competent in the delivery of nursing care, the need to train to understand and be able to function as a leader is fundamental to the identity of the twenty-first-century nurse. You are encouraged, therefore, not only to engage with the written content of the book, but also to undertake the activities (described in more detail below). The activities are integral to the learning from this book, and you should keep a written record of what you do to engage with them and what you find out as a result.

Who should read the book?

You should read this book if you have, or aspire to have, some element of leadership in the workplace. This applies equally to student nurses, trained nurses, associate nurses and other professionals working in the health and social care arena.

What is it about?

This book focuses on the attitudes, values and practices which serve to make for good leadership and management. Throughout the book the focus is on challenging the reader to adopt an approach to leadership and management which is focused on the human elements of the role. Readers are prompted to think about the ideals which brought them into nursing practice in the first place and consider how these might apply to what they do as potential and actual leaders or managers of people.

Why is it important?

This book is important for you because it brings together many of the elements of nursing leadership which you need to understand both now, as you lead other less-experienced students, associate nurses and healthcare support workers, and in the future as you become responsible for managing shifts, teams and organisations. Like nursing, leadership is both an art and a science and like nursing, leadership requires you to engage with lifelong learning in order to develop your abilities to practise it.

The special importance of this book is that it is grounded in the learning and development of the author, who has been a practising nurse and a leader. The book itself contains case studies and anecdotes from a variety of areas of practice which identify and demystify nurse leadership.

How is it structured?

The format of the book reflects the way in which we see the need for students to think about what it means to be led, to work in a team and to lead and manage development. The individual chapters can be read and understood on their own, but read together they help form a coherent picture of what good leadership and management practice look like.

Chapter 1, *Experience of management and leadership*, highlights the importance of remembering and understanding what it means to be led and what this might mean for the way in which you subsequently choose to lead.

Chapter 2, *Frameworks for management and leadership*, identifies and examines some theories of leadership and management and their interconnectedness. This provides a solid foundation for the rest of the book.

Chapter 3, *Teams and teamwork*, identifies what teams are, why they exist and how they can work better toward their common goals. Then Chapter 4, *Working with individuals in teams*, introduces the roles and responsibilities of individuals within teams, and issues such as recruitment and delegation.

In Chapter 5, *Conflict management and negotiation skills*, the different personality types that may operate within teams are described, and ways of managing conflict within the team and other settings are explored. Following this, Chapter 6, *Coaching, mentoring and clinical supervision*, investigates the role of the leader or manager in supporting team members.

Chapter 7, *Improving care and change management*, presents theories which may underpin leadership practice in relationship to the instigation and management of change, while Chapter 8, *Creating a learning environment*, considers the value of understanding the culture within which teams work and the impact this may have on the successful working of the team.

In Chapter 9, *Developing confidence as a manager and leader*, some of the tasks and roles undertaken by the leader or manager are laid bare. The chapter goes on to look at how these might be used to develop certainty in what they do for the developing leader.

NMC Standards of Proficiency

This edition refers to the NMC's *Future Nurse: Standards of Proficiency for Registered Nurses* (NMC, 2018a) as they pertain to your development as a nurse, although its content is not narrowly defined by these standards.

Activities

The activities contained within each chapter form an integral part of the learning and development strategy for that chapter. You will get the most benefit from each chapter if you engage fully with the activities, and in the order they are presented. The activities are designed to help illustrate the nature and reality of some of the theory presented and to bring to life some of the situations, scenarios and associated skills and competences described. Some of the activities require you to seek out new information and new experiences; engagement with this process adds not only to you developing your understanding of the theory underpinning good leadership and management practice, but also to developing the skills and competences to apply them in practice.

Reflection on the chapter content and on the activities is an important and integral part of the process of the student nurse's development as a leader of people. Some activities require you to come to a decision or understanding for yourself, while others have suggested answers presented at the end of the chapter. You should consider each activity for yourself before reading the suggested answers so you can come to an understanding of your own level of understanding of the content of the chapter as well as your own personal and professional development.

Other features

The text includes case studies and scenarios, research summaries and the necessary theory. There is a glossary of terms at the end of the book. Glossary entries will be in bold type the first time they appear in any chapter.

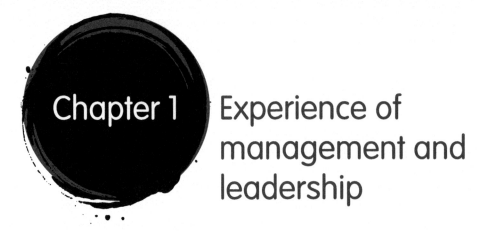

Chapter 1   Experience of management and leadership

Platform 5: Leading and managing nursing care and working in teams

Registered nurses provide leadership by acting as a role model for best practice in the delivery of nursing care. They are responsible for managing nursing care and are accountable for the appropriate delegation and supervision of care provided by others in the team including lay carers. They play an active and equal role in the interdisciplinary team, collaborating and communicating effectively with a range of colleagues.

At the point of registration, the registered nurse will be able to:

5.4   demonstrate an understanding of the roles, responsibilities and scope of practice of all members of the nursing and interdisciplinary team and how to make best use of the contributions of others involved in providing care.

Platform 7: Coordinating care

Registered nurses play a leadership role in coordinating and managing the complex nursing and integrated care needs of people at any stage of their lives, across a range of organisations and settings. They contribute to processes of organisational change through an awareness of local and national policies.

At the point of registration, the registered nurse will be able to:

7.7   understand how to monitor and evaluate the quality of people's experience of complex care.

Chapter aims

After reading this chapter, you will be able to:

- identify some of the values which underpin nursing and nurse leadership and management;
- reflect on and understand how the experience of being led affects the ways in which we choose to lead and manage in nursing;
- comment on the importance of leadership and management in nursing;
- begin to create a coherent picture of what leadership and management structures in nursing look like.

Introduction

The purpose of this chapter is to increase your awareness of the personal and professional values that influence how managers and leaders should behave. The chapter will both challenge and reinforce some of the assumptions you hold about the ways in which leaders and managers function.

Our **values** and assumptions about leadership and management are largely derived from our experiences of leading and managing, and of being led and managed. They will therefore reflect our personal interpretation of what happened during the process. At the start of any quest to understand leadership and management, it is important to understand ourselves and our motivations. Only in this way can we hope to understand the context of leadership and management and the behaviours and motivations of those we seek to lead.

As well as exploring the context of values in relation to leadership and management, this chapter examines some characteristics of leaders and managers. These reflect the characteristics leadership and management theorists believe good managers and leaders should portray, including their personality traits. After examining these characteristics, you will be encouraged to formulate a picture of how you believe good leaders or managers should behave, and the essential qualities they should exhibit within the nursing context.

Chapter 2 gives a more detailed discussion of theories and frameworks for leadership and management, and how they can meet the challenges of twenty-first-century nursing.

This chapter considers why leadership and management matter to nursing practice, now and in the future, and how an understanding of them can contribute to your personal and professional development. We will examine this issue in the context of some of the findings of the Francis report (2013), which examined serious failures in care.

Toward the end of the chapter, some of the reasons for the existence of different leadership and management roles in nursing are introduced and discussed. You are invited to collect data on the nursing structures where you work and consider how these impact on the work you and your colleagues do.

Understanding context and values

Our ideas and opinions about good leadership and management are coloured by personal experiences of leadership and management, whether we are managers, leaders or team members. The assumptions we have about management and leadership styles and behaviours are also affected by our understanding of the motivations behind the management and leadership styles we adopt or see adopted. The inability to understand why a certain approach to management or leadership has been adopted can lead to misconceptions and misunderstandings; this is something an awareness of the context of nurse leadership and management allows us to see beyond. Sometimes this context is better developed as we gain more experiences as nurses and reflect thoughtfully on these.

Activity 1.1   Reflection

When you first came into nursing, or care, and went into practice for the first time, how did you feel about the efforts made by the staff to get frail, elderly patients to engage in self-care (for example, encouraging them to get out of bed in the morning and get washed and dressed)? Now you understand a bit more about the purpose and nature of nursing, have you changed your view? Why?

There are some possible answers and thoughts at the end of the chapter.

Understanding why something is done in a particular way in each situation allows us to understand the context of an action in the clinical setting. As shown in Activity 1.1, a developing understanding of the nature of nursing and what it means to nurse helps us to make sense of the world of work and the roles in which we find ourselves. In this case, the less-experienced practitioner may consider efforts to engage elderly patients in their care as cruel or lazy, while more experience lets you see enablement and rehabilitation as fundamental aspects of the role of the nurse. The same is true of leadership and management, where actions taken out of context may appear to be wrong. For example, preventing a carer from working because they have not completed their moving and handling training could be regarded as callous, but to a manager, the need for the training relates to the safety of the patients, the carer, other team members and the wider organisation.

One of the enduring difficulties for student nurses can be to understand the provision of care beyond the individual. Often the context of nursing management and leadership is about achieving the best outcomes on a regular, recurring and equitable basis for the many. The need to achieve good outcomes for the many may help us to understand the context of a management or leadership style we see before us (as in the moving and handling training example). This view is one which can only develop if we are willing and able to question and reflect on the leadership and management practices we see around us.

Case study: The newly qualified nurse

Julius is a newly qualified staff nurse working on a busy cardiology ward. Julius is irritated by the apparent inactivity of the ward sister Deirdre, who spends vast amounts of time in the office doing what, to him, appears to be nothing instead of providing patient care. Julius confronts Deirdre about the lack of time she spends on the ward and suggests that much of the time she is doing nothing of value while she is 'hiding away' in her office.

(Continued)

(Continued)

Deirdre understands the point Julius is making and is wise enough to appreciate that his frustrations arise not out of malice toward her but because of his inexperience and lack of understanding of what it takes to keep a busy ward functioning smoothly. Deirdre takes Julius into her office and shows him some of the tasks she must perform on a regular basis, which include writing the duty roster, completing staff appraisals, entering patient dependency scores onto a monitoring database and liaising with other professionals both in the hospital and externally.

Deirdre explains to Julius that she, too, is frustrated by the lack of time she has to provide care: that, she explains, is after all why she came into nursing. But she also understands her role now is less about providing care and more about facilitating the delivery of care. Deirdre explains she achieves this through supporting the staff on the ward to improve, using appraisals and accessing appropriate education and development; rostering to allow for a good work–life balance; and recording the level of dependency of the patients and the stock requirements. She explains she sees her role as supporting the staff to care for the patients, including engaging with other professionals to get the input patients need. If she did not do the necessary tasks there would be chaos, and patient care would be impacted.

Julius concedes he had not looked at things in this way and he needed to understand the wider context before criticising.

This example demonstrates that one of the necessary qualities of a good manager or leader is the ability to see the bigger picture and anticipate and plan what the team will be doing and how they will do it. Leadership and management are, therefore, as much forward-looking activities as about managing what is happening in the here and now. One of the characteristics of good managers or leaders is understanding what it is they want to achieve and being able to communicate this, and perhaps effectively delegating to the team. This relates well to Platform 5 'Leading and managing nursing care and working in teams', outcome 5.4, stated at the start of the chapter as: *demonstrate an understanding of the roles, responsibilities and scope of practice of all members of the nursing and interdisciplinary team and how to make best use of the contributions of others involved in providing care.* Julius has some work to do to be able to meet this outcome, but that is OK. He has time to grow into the role.

We should remember at this stage that some of the most important things that motivate us as nurses to achieve our goals are our values. Before we explore the context of nursing leadership and management further, let's stop for a moment to reflect on the values we have as humans, nurses, leaders or managers and see what impact they might have on leadership and management in nursing.

It is not at all easy to state exactly what values are. A cursory search on the internet for values of caring throws up scores of words, all of which may have relevance to nursing, but none of which explain what they are. Various descriptions include reference to dignity, privacy, best interests, moral duties, likes and preferences.

Concept summary: Human values

One of the most widely cited definitions of values, and one which has resonance with nurse leadership, is the definition by Schwartz (1994, p20), who says that a value is *a belief pertaining to desirable end states or modes of conduct that transcends specific situations; guides selection or evaluation of behavior, people, and events; and is ordered by the importance relative to other values to form a system of value priorities.*

The notable elements of the definition by Schwartz are that values relate to:

- achieving a good outcome;
- something more important than individual situations;
- how we ought to behave;
- what we ought to look for in the behaviour of others;
- how events ought to be managed;
- ways in which we might prioritise how we use our time and effort.

In essence, the suggestion here is that our values should be at the centre of everything we do, both as a guide to how we act as well as what it is we act upon. The additional issue for leaders and managers is, of course, that they need to role model these values to those they lead.

Evidently, within the case study above, Deirdre had not forgotten the values that took her into nursing in the first place. What had changed for Deirdre as she moved from a clinical role to a more managerial post was simply the way in which these values could express themselves. To develop continually as nurses, leaders and managers, it is important not only that we question our values from time to time, but that we are also able to express what these values are and refine them in discussion with our colleagues.

Activity 1.2 Decision-making

Take some time to think about the values you have as a nurse. Now think about how these values show themselves in the ways in which you act when in the clinical setting. Next time you are in practice, ask your team leader or ward manager what values they hold and how they think they express them in practice. Now compare the lists, looking for areas of overlap and areas of difference. What do you notice about the similarities and differences between your list of values and corresponding actions and the leader's values and actions?

There are some possible answers and thoughts at the end of the chapter.

What is clear about the values of practising nurses, ward managers and more senior nursing staff is they should, and to a great extent do, share similar values and goals. These values will relate to things like care, maintaining and promoting dignity and doing good. You should not mistake them for political or other opinions, which may differ widely even among a group of nurses who work together. The role of the leader or manager should be to facilitate the team in achieving these values and goals. Evidently, where there are differences in the values and goals of the team and the team leader, then difficulties will arise. When nurses or nurse leaders forget what their values are, then they will lose sight of what it is they are trying to achieve.

Sometimes it is hard to know what exactly our values are, or the limits to which they can be stretched. One method for understanding our values as potential leaders or managers is to ask ourselves hypothetical questions, the answers to which can be searching and difficult for us. The answers enable us, however, to understand what sort of people we are and what motivates us as humans, nurses and managers. Understanding our own values and underlying motivations will then tell us something about what is likely to motivate and guide the actions of those that may be called upon to lead. You might also quite simply be able to reflect on situations where you have acted in one way and then spent some time regretting it because 'that is not who I am' – this, 'who am I?' is a useful tool for understanding what motivates us and makes us who we are, in other words our values.

Scenario 1.1: Doing the right thing

Imagine you are working in a nursing home on nights. You are tired, having already worked six shifts in a row. One of the residents, Jane, who is in her late 80s, has been in the home for some time following a stroke. Jane needs to be turned 4-hourly to avoid her developing pressure sores, but you and the nurse you are working with decide to turn her just once over the 12-hour shift. You justify this to yourselves by saying this avoids disturbing her sleep and it also protects your backs. At the end of the shift, you turn her and record in her notes that you have done so 4-hourly throughout the night. She has not developed a pressure sore, so what is the harm?

Now consider this: you turn her at the end of the night and discover that a small area has broken down on her left hip. Is this your fault? If the manager asks if you have turned her 4-hourly, as stated in the care plan, what will you say? You could say you turned her 4-hourly – this would not change anything for Jane, but would make your life easier.

Alternatively, you go to turn her at the end of the night shift only to discover that she has died some time during the night. She has been dead for a while judging from how cold she is and the blood that is pooling on the side she was lying on. You know you can just claim that you found her earlier in the night and prepare her body quickly before the day staff come in to work. Surely this will not change anything; no one will be hurt, will they?

Which, if any, of these scenarios are acceptable? Does the blame attached to any of them change because of the outcome? What does your choice of actions say about you? What values are being displayed here? How do they compare with the values you expressed in Activity 1.2?

There are some possible answers and thoughts at the end of the chapter.

Examining examples such as this enables us to see the bigger picture. They also help us to increase our awareness of our own values. In part, our values will be mirrored in the sort of person we are and how we see the world in general, but they will also shape the way in which the world sees us. Of course, it might be equally bad if a nurse were to follow policy and procedure blindly, with no thought about the consequences. In this scenario, as in many leadership and management situations, deviating from what we know to be right (i.e. ignoring our values) can have dire consequences for those we care for and for us, both as nurses and humans, as well as for the people we work with.

Scenario 1.2: Being clear

You are working on a medical admissions unit and have asked a colleague, Emma, to go round and do the observations. She takes the temperature, pulse and blood pressure of every patient on the unit, as asked. About an hour later you ask if all the observations were OK. Emma replies that the woman in the first bed had a temperature of 39°C. You ask why she had not informed you of this immediately. She replies that it was her job to do the observations as you asked, and that is what she has done.

What does this scenario tell you about managing and leading people in the clinical setting? What does this tell you about the need to understand what we do and why? Is there a place for understanding values of care in this scenario?

There are some possible answers and thoughts at the end of the chapter.

By now you should have developed a clear picture of the values you believe underpin what you do as a student nurse or nurse. You may also have some insight into the values of those around you and the impact working among other nurses has on the development of your own values. It is important to understand that, for leaders or managers to be effective, there is a requirement for there to be some degree of overlap between their values and the values of their team. The team must be aware of this and where this is not the case, leaders must work to ensure it happens (Giddens, 2018). Put simply, to lead you need people to follow and followers need to want to follow; people will more readily follow those whose values they share.

What happens when values are forgotten?

Health and social care teams are made up of collections of people working together to achieve a common task. This common task, as we have seen, requires that the values of the individuals involved in the care align to some extent; otherwise they would be working in opposition to, rather than with, each other. One of the challenges of modern healthcare is that our values can get lost among all the tasks we have to undertake, and our attention may be drawn instead to achieving goals and targets.

When nurses, or indeed any care staff, forget the values that should be driving their work, this has an impact on the culture they work in and this culture ultimately impacts on the care they give.

The following extract is taken from the Francis *Report of the Mid Staffordshire NHS Foundation Trust Public Inquiry* (2013):

> *The negative aspects of culture in the system were identified as including:*
> - *a lack of openness to criticism*
> - *a lack of consideration for patients*
> - *defensiveness*
> - *looking inwards, not outwards*
> - *secrecy*
> - *misplaced assumptions about the judgements and actions of others*
> - *an acceptance of poor standards*
> - *a failure to put the patient first in everything that is done.*
>
> *It cannot be suggested that all these characteristics are present everywhere in the system all of the time, far from it, but their existence anywhere means that there is an insufficiently shared positive culture.*
>
> (Francis, 2013, p65)

What is being identified here is not a list of issues with the organisation, but a list of issues which arise because the collective values of the people in the organisation have become secondary to other issues. If we take each of the bullet points in turn, we can see each one represents a *value* which is not being exercised:

- competence;
- compassion;
- thankfulness;
- mindfulness;
- openness;
- trust;
- principles;
- care.

The report continues:

> *To change that, there needs to be a relentless focus on the patient's interests and the obligation to keep patients safe and protected from substandard care. This means that the patient must be first in everything that is done: there must be no tolerance of substandard care; frontline staff must be empowered with responsibility and freedom to act in this way under strong and stable leadership in stable organisations.*

To achieve this does not require radical reorganisation but re-emphasis of what is truly important:

- *emphasis on and commitment to common values throughout the system by all within it.*

(Francis, 2013, p66)

The Francis report had a major impact on the way in which care is delivered in the UK, not because what happened at Mid Staffordshire was unique (it probably wasn't), but because it reminded care professionals and politicians alike that, once managers impose the wrong sorts of *values* and *targets* on care professionals, then values of care can easily be forgotten. Again, the message is about having values which are common to leaders, managers and staff.

The coronavirus pandemic which affected most of the world throughout 2020 and 2021 has highlighted some collective emotions and behaviours which can be understood as relating to values. Grint (2020) identifies how the common enemy at times like this is the virus and how there is no time for nationalistic values, but only for human ones. Among the values Grint (2020) identifies is the need to support people who need it. There have been countless examples during the pandemic, both within nursing and in the wider population.

To become an effective leader or manager of people, we first must know ourselves and our values, as well as having some insight into how others see us and how they interpret the way in which we display our values. Part of leadership or management is presentation of self to others and encouraging others to follow our lead by behaving in ways and displaying values that others admire and can identify with – creating a situation where others wish to follow. A leader without followers is just a person working alone!

How we see ourselves and others see us

To understand how we see ourselves and how this compares to how others see us, it is worth looking at the work of Joseph Luft and Harry Ingham, whose Johari window illustrates the point about what we know about ourselves and what others know about us.

What the Johari window allows us to see is how much of the perceptions and knowledge we have about ourselves is also seen and shared by others:

- The open/free area refers to what we know about ourselves and what is also known by other people – it is our public face.
- The blind area is the area of our personality we are blind to but which others can see – our blind spot.
- The hidden area is what we know about ourselves but we keep hidden from others, sometimes called the 'avoided self' or 'facade'.
- The unknown area refers to what is unknown both to ourselves and to others (which can be regarded as an area for potential development and self-exploration).

What is interesting about this model is it shows us there is great potential for us to lack understanding of ourselves as much as there is potential for other people not to understand us. To some extent, we can manage the view others have of us by allowing them to see what we want them to see and by managing our behaviours at work and in our private lives. On the other hand, people are often aware of issues with our values and personality that we are sometimes aware of and sometimes not.

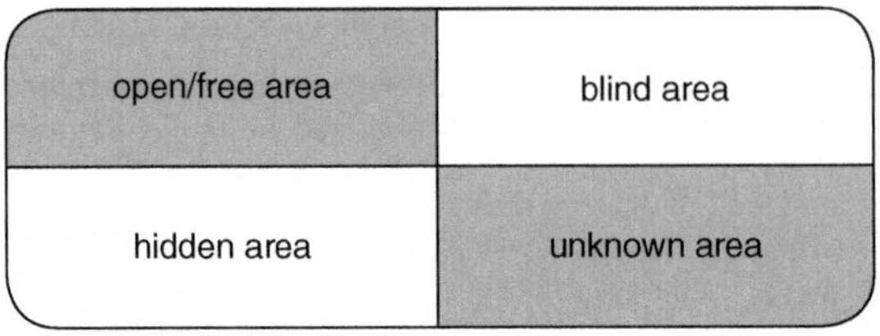

Figure 1.1   The Johari window

Source: Adapted from Luft and Ingham (1955), p10.

Being able to adapt who we are and how we behave at work is part of the process of socialising to be both a nurse and a member of society. By being aware of our values and acting upon them we allow ourselves the ability to become someone we want to become and potentially to develop the traits that will help us to develop as a person, a nurse and, over time, as a manager or leader.

Activity 1.3   Communication

In order to get some idea of how your view of yourself is similar to, or differs from, that of other people, undertake the following exercise which may tell you something about how you communicate with and are perceived by other people. Choose a colour which you think describes what sort of person you believe yourself to be and write down why you think the colour applies to you and how it represents the facets of your personality. Ask several people you know to choose a colour which describes what sort of person you are and ask them to explain their choice. Include fellow students, lecturers, practice assessors and other people you work with. Write the choices and reasons down and compare them for similarities and differences. Assign the responses to the various boxes of the Johari window and consider what this says about how your perception of self concurs or contrasts with the views of others.

Since this is based on your own thoughts and reflections, there is no specimen answer at the end of the chapter.

Activity 1.3 will help you to see that sometimes people see good and sometimes bad things about us which we may or may not see for ourselves. Their overall impression of us may be quite different from who we think we are and the person we think we are portraying. You will also notice that different people interpret elements of your personality in divergent ways.

The lesson for would-be leaders is to learn to change the negatives we can change and to manage the areas of our personality we cannot. You should also be prepared to take onboard positive insights and use these to continue to improve your relationships with others. One of the main functions of a leader and manager is the development of others; however, the failure to develop oneself does not create the confidence in others that you know what you are doing in this regard.

What are the characteristics of a good leader or manager?

What makes a good leader or manager has been explored by many theorists and academics over the years. Some of the early theorists identified characteristics such as physical size, strength and 'presence' (Wright, 1996). Other characteristics and traits that have been favoured include intelligence, personality type such as extroversion, and **charisma** and other interpersonal skills.

Certainly, it is true that being **charismatic** and intelligent helps with the processing of ideas and when communicating with others. But, as we have seen above, there must be more to being a good nurse, good leader or good manager than these qualities alone. Sometimes extreme examples allow us to see things that are perhaps not clear to us in the day-to-day process of being managed or led.

Activity 1.4   Reflection

Reflect on some of the leadership you saw both in the UK and internationally during the coronavirus pandemic. Consider some of the key players in the UK and not only their role, but also the way in which their message came across and the faith people had in what they said. You might think of politicians like Boris Johnson, Nicola Sturgeon, Rishi Sunak and Matt Hancock. What, if any, faith did you have in what they said and why? How did they compare, during the crisis, to international political figures such as Donald Trump, Vladimir Putin or Emmanuel Macron? How do you feel about their approach to managing coronavirus and what shapes your opinion of them?

Perhaps also consider the teams of specialists who have informed the country throughout the coronavirus; people like Professors Chris Whitty and Jonathan Van-Tam and Dr Jenny Harries. What sort of leadership do you think they have shown? What is the basis of this leadership and how do you feel about their approach to it?

There are some possible answers and thoughts at the end of the chapter.

What we can see about the leaders in Activity 1.4, and what perhaps others know about some of them that they do not see for themselves, is the leaders we admire have a vision of something better for the people they lead. In the case of the national coronavirus leadership teams, this may have been the ability to talk about a shared way forward, about common purpose and the generation of a sense of belonging. Conversely, we also saw when politicians and political figures have acted in ways which did not reflect the common good, how their inability to act as they speak has led to widespread apolitical condemnation. The pursuit of these values and the veracity with which they pursued them give us a clue as to one other quality we might admire in a leader: **integrity** (Barr and Dowding, 2019). In this sense, integrity may be understood as acting in a manner that reflects the values, ethics and morals that an individual believes to be important.

Integrity alone is not enough, however. Historical leaders like Hitler and Stalin perhaps believed in what they were doing; in that sense they had integrity. What is interesting about what they believed and what they set out to achieve is that it was often more about achieving power for themselves than it was about achieving what was right or something that benefits others.

What is missing, therefore, is an understanding about what this integrity and leadership should be aimed at achieving. Staff look to their nurse leaders for coaching and guidance (Manges et al., 2017) and the purpose of teams is to get a job of work done, increasing organisational productivity (Tamunomiebi and Uhuru, 2018). In nursing, this job is about providing care for others in a manner that reflects the positive values we hold as humans and as nurses. For a nurse leader or manager, therefore, integrity of action means leading, managing and coaching in a manner that reflects the values of care which are part of what being a nurse is about and which you have identified for yourself in Activity 1.2.

Activity 1.5   Reflection

Take the time now to reflect on the people you have been led by in your life and consider what was either good or bad about their behaviours and way of interacting with you and others. What values did they show and what caused you to either admire or disapprove of them? Common examples might be a teacher, a lecturer or a sports coach.

Since this is based on your own observations there is no specimen answer at the end of the chapter.

So far in this chapter we have seen that being a good leader or manager in nursing is about the expression of the same values of care that being a good nurse requires. What changes when one moves from being a nurse to a nurse leader or manager is the way in which these values are expressed through what we do and how we behave. The consistency of the values between nursing and nurse leadership/management demonstrates integrity – especially when these are expressed in the same individual on their journey from team worker to team leader and beyond. It is a sad fact that those nurse leaders and managers who we see losing sight of their values are the ones we least admire. Salvage and White (2019) point out how the most outstanding of nurse leaders maintain the ability to retain a moral compass which guides their actions at both a micro and a macro level.

The report into the failings at the Mid Staffordshire Hospital identified poor leadership coupled with clinical staff *accepting standards of care … that should not have been tolerated* (Clews, 2010). The collective failing here was that clinically trained managers did not support their staff as well as they might have and the managers and leaders, as well as their staff, allowed standards of care to slip below a level reflective of the true *values* of nursing.

One of the challenges of this book is for you to recognise and acknowledge the values you have as a nursing student and to think about how you will continue to exercise these values throughout your nursing career.

Structures of nurse leadership

What we have not discussed so far are the structures that relate to the exercise of leadership and management. A manager occupies a formal role. The role of the manager is conferred upon the individual by an organisation and its staff are responsible to the manager by virtue of their contract of employment with the organisation – often called **legitimate power** (first identified by French and Raven in 1960). How these lines of responsibility are created and what they mean in practice should be clearer after the next activity.

Activity 1.6   Reflection

To understand the lines of responsibility that form part of a contract, look at the handbook for the university programme you are on. There will be clear guidelines about some things you can and cannot do as a university student. There will be identified individuals to whom you would have to answer if you break these rules. This forms part of your contract with the university and ultimately with the NMC in relation to the fitness to practise criteria.

Alternatively, if you have a contract of employment, you may notice it identifies the person to whom you are responsible, usually a line manager (like the ward sister) and to whom you are accountable within the organisation (often the nursing director).

As this is based on your own observations there is no specimen answer at the end of the chapter.

Managerial power and responsibility, as you can see from Activity 1.6, are therefore formalised within the contract of employment or training. They are validated since we choose to submit to these contracts of our own free will, usually because they will confer some benefit on us (in the case of a job, being paid and in the case of being a student nurse, in gaining a qualification). Similarly, as nurses, we agree to be bound by *The Code* and other regulations pertaining to nursing (NMC, 2018b).

Within most organisations there are several managers at different levels who have different responsibilities. These managers report to a more senior manager who, in turn, reports to more senior management. Such structures are formalised and are usually created to allow for the overseeing of the functions of the organisation. Each tier within the system of management should be aware of their responsibilities and the limits of their powers in fulfilling the tasks associated with these roles. It is often helpful for novice nurses to have some idea of what the structure of the organisation they work in looks like.

In Chapter 8 we consider cultures of care; you may find it useful to look up Charles Handy's work (1994) on cultures to inform your thinking about the formal and informal management structures which can exist in health and social care.

Activity 1.7   Evidence-based practice and research

Try to find out something about the management structure in the hospital, community team, hospice or care home in which you are placed. There may be a diagram that shows the relative management positions (sometimes called an organogram). Then try to find out what the main responsibilities are of the people in the various roles you have identified. You might also like to do something similar for a ward or other practice area so you can get an overview of who is responsible for what.

As this is based on your own observation there is no specimen answer at the end of the chapter.

We can see that being a manager is a formalised role that is conferred by position within an organisation. Being a leader, on the other hand, may or may not be the result of position within a team or organisation. How can this be?

As we will see elsewhere in the book, leadership is in many instances one of the roles of a manager. Think about the managers in the areas where you have worked who as well as managing the unit also lead the team. Think also about the areas where you have worked where individuals occupying junior roles in a team appear to exercise leadership. Sometimes, then, the leadership function is one of the roles of the manager, while on other occasions something else is happening.

How then do some non-managers function as leaders? Essentially there are three answers to this question. First, some leaders, such as team leaders, are designated leaders because they are more experienced than the other staff or they hold a higher, non-management grade. They exercise the power of leadership also through virtue of the formal position they hold and the delegation of certain duties from their line manager. In this respect the power they exercise comes from the person who has delegated it to them and is legitimate power. The leadership roles within such an arrangement are therefore legitimised because they represent a choice on the part of the people who are led by these elected, or contractual, leaders.

Second, other leaders exercise leadership in relation to specific projects or responsibilities within the team. For example, in many teams there are link nurses with responsibility for areas such as diabetes care, wound management or infection control. Again, their power to act as leaders is, in part, conferred by the role they are asked to play in the team and is delegated from the team manager. The other reason they are a leader in their particular area is because they have specialist knowledge. In this situation a good leader will share the information the team needs to know to get the job done effectively and safely – a bad leader will not! Clearly, then, one of the characteristics of a leader is information management and good communication.

Third, there are those people who lead by virtue of their character. These charismatic individuals are the sort of people others like and respond to. They can motivate others and get the team to follow them by virtue of who they are. They have a compelling vision of what should be done and how and have a conviction and surety about them which encourages others to follow their lead. They have what is often called emotional intelligence, which is discussed later in the book, and which others in the team warm to as they feel respected, cared for and appreciated (Morsiani et al., 2017). They may not be in positions of formal power, but perhaps they have knowledge and/or good communication skills that single them out as people others like to follow.

Case study: The new nursing sister

Eileen is a newly appointed sister on the dialysis unit of a busy general hospital. Eileen is liked by all the staff but has rapidly built up a reputation for being quite disorganised. When she is in charge of the shift, things go wrong. She gets side-tracked by small details and disappears for long periods of time to sort out seemingly minor issues.

Karen is a healthcare assistant who has worked in the dialysis unit for many years. Karen is familiar with the routine and is able to cope with most situations that arise. Karen often takes charge of the unit, even when Eileen is there. She co-ordinates the workload, makes telephone calls and arranges transport. Karen uses her connections and the relationships she has built up over the years to get things done.

What we can see in this case study is that, even within an essentially quite hierarchical structure, leadership can be found at all levels of the team. In this example there is a real danger that Eileen, who has legitimate power, will lose control of the unit and Karen, who has charismatic power, might overstep her own competence, role and responsibilities. One of the issues that arises out of this scenario is accountability. Eileen, as a registered nurse, is accountable for what she does as well as the actions of her team, especially the untrained members – including Karen. Karen as a care assistant is not accountable for her actions in the same way, but is responsible to her employer (actually, Eileen) for what she does.

In this scenario, the power which Karen exercises is not strictly speaking legitimate. As with all members of the team, she has roles and responsibilities for which she may need to exercise the power given to her by virtue of her position. It may be that Karen has the power to order stores and perhaps organise transport, but these are subject to the need to recognise the roles and responsibilities of other members of the team, who may need support in developing the skills necessary for them to operate effectively.

It may be argued, therefore, that the leadership that Karen exercises is, in this instance, a bad thing. Karen is perhaps motivated to get the immediate job done, but perhaps misses some of the bigger-picture issues, such as the quality of the dialysis, that she is not in a position to understand. Because Karen takes over the day-to-day running of the unit, she is also both undermining Eileen and preventing her from developing into her new role. While in the short term this might appear to work, it is not a long-term solution; remember how we said that the manager needs to see the micro and the macro in any situation.

Activity 1.8   Reflection

Take some time to think about the implications of this case study. Have you seen similar situations? If so, what were the positive aspects for the team and what were the negative ones? How did the role reversal affect you and other members of the immediate team?

There are some possible answers and thoughts at the end of the chapter.

So, we have seen that leadership and management within nursing can be broken down into many levels, from the most senior member of the nursing team right through to the most junior, and the qualities that make a good leader can be present at all levels. We have also seen that some managers fail to lead and that some leaders do not really have the formal position or power to do so.

Leading and managing: the policy context

What we do as nurses, and what nurse managers and leaders do, occurs within a healthcare context and is subject to policy, procedure and guidelines. If leadership or management is about leading or managing a team to achieve certain outcomes, and within healthcare these outcomes are derived from policy and guidelines, then there is a need for nurse leaders and managers not only to be aware of what the guidelines are but also to act on them and ensure their team acts on them too.

Historically the caring professions had a great deal of autonomy over the ways in which they worked. In the past they set the standards by which their work was to be measured and audited and decided on clinical and non-clinical priorities. More recently, most notably following the policies of the Thatcher government and subsequently New Labour, clinical priority setting and the standards for care have been determined more centrally through government policy via agencies such as the National Institute for Health and Care Excellence (NICE) or via nationally drawn-up structures for care, such as the National Service Frameworks. So, part of the role of nurse leaders or managers will be having the ability to lead or manage their team through the change process to achieve the outcomes of care determined from outside the team (see Chapter 8).

During the COVID-19 pandemic, the creation, publication and adoption of policies became more visible to the public than ever. We saw, for example, visiting policies in hospitals and care homes, not only imposed centrally, but also subjected to public scrutiny and critique. Such times have called for nurse leaders to step up and represent their organisations' responses to these public policies.

As well as general policy and guidelines in health and social care, nurses are subject to policy and guidance from our professional body, the NMC. To understand the context of leadership and management in nursing from the point of view of the NMC, it is worth familiarising yourself with the standards and educational outcomes identified at the start of each chapter and asking yourself how these apply within the context of each chapter. You may also wish to look at and reflect on how these ideas reflect the issues identified within other NMC documentation, including *The Code* (NMC, 2018b). Most especially, this chapter has highlighted the need for a nurse leader to be *an accountable professional* as demonstrated in Platform 1 where the nurse has to: *understand and act in accordance with the Code (2018b): Professional standards of practice and behaviour for nurses, midwives and nursing associates and fulfil all registration requirements.*

In this chapter we have discussed some of the values that underpin nursing practice, as well as leadership and management characteristics of the good nurse leader/manager. These characteristics translate well from both the code of professional conduct and the education proficiencies identified at the start of the chapter. What they validate is the core message of the chapter: to become a good leader or manager of nurses it is important to remain grounded in the values, beliefs and behaviours that guide professional nursing practice.

Think of the leadership function this way: policy and guidelines determine what we do; at a local level these may be seen as mission or vision statements, while how we deliver care and how we behave generally is an expression of our values. Policy and guidelines provide the what, values provide the how.

Chapter summary

Rather than launch straight into a discussion about the nature of leadership and management in nursing, this chapter has sought to identify some of the values, beliefs and behaviours that might be associated with becoming a good nurse leader or manager. These characteristics have been compared and contrasted with some of the values that underpin being a good nurse. There is an explicit challenge here for you to identify and confront the values you have as a nurse, a nursing student, a team member and a leader.

In some part this challenge has been posed by reference to some of the shortcomings identified in the Francis report. While the failings at Mid Staffordshire NHS Trust are useful as a benchmark of what can go wrong, they are exactly that; a benchmark. They should not be considered as merely a footnote in history but should be seen as a salutary lesson in what could easily happen anywhere when nurses and other care professionals neglect their values.

An understanding of the context of care and of ourselves is an important first step on the road to becoming a competent leader of nurses; failure to understand what motivates us as individuals lays us open to external criticism. Furthermore, some of the skills and values we develop as nurses in clinical practice will translate well into leadership and management roles. It is never too soon for student nurses to think about what type of leader/manager they want to be and to look around them for suitable role models to guide their development.

Activities: Brief outline answers

Activity 1.1 Reflection (p7)

This reflection is not about understanding the rehabilitation of the elderly as such; it is about understanding context. As a new nurse you may consider asking people to undertake their own care as lazy nursing, because you consider nursing as a caring profession that does things for people. As you understand the nature of care better, you will see the same scenario in a different light or context, as you understand that encouraging self-care is about helping people address their care deficits and achieve the activities of daily living for themselves.

Activity 1.2 Decision-making (p9)

What you will notice is that the basic values of caring, moral behaviour, putting others before self, protection of rights, autonomy and dignity are common to both lists. What will be different is that the leader will attempt to achieve these aims through the way in which they lead. This will include acting as a role model and promoting the welfare of the team who, in turn, are expected to support these values one-to-one with patients and clients (Salmela et al., 2017). If you are still struggling to think about what your values are, try some of the words above or choose some from this list: accountability, accuracy, calmness, commitment, decisiveness, fairness, honesty, integrity, justice, openness, reliability, team work or truthfulness.

Scenario 1.1 Doing the right thing (p10)

We hope you found none of these scenarios acceptable. On each occasion, regardless of the outcome, the choice being made was to avoid your duty to Jane to protect her from potential further physical harm. The values displayed here are self-regarding and not other-regarding and are against everything that is to be found in *The Code* (NMC, 2018b). At best, the scenario demonstrates lies being told and at worst a dereliction of the duty of care, leading to harm to the patient. Some people might argue that, as no harm ensued, the first scenario might be all right, but the consequences that *could* accrue (as seen later in the scenario) show this to be wrong, regardless of any arguments about duty and outcomes. Of course, the precedent in your behaviour and that of the colleague involved may well lead to further harm being done to other patients at a later date, even if you 'got away with it' this time.

Scenario 1.2 Being clear (p11)

This scenario suggests that as a manager or leader it is important not only to have team members who do what they are asked, but also that they understand the purpose of what they are doing. There is a clear need here for the nurse to understand that doing observations is not enough in itself; it is acting on what is found that is important. The value which should drive the undertaking of such tasks is **person-centred** care, which requires that nurses not only undertake a task, but that they think about what it means for the patient or client.

Activity 1.4 Reflection (p15)

No matter what your political leanings it would be hard to deny that being a politician during the time of the coronavirus pandemic has been challenging. Some of the issues you think about in relation to the politicians may include their ability to be open and honest. Perhaps, during the crisis, they have managed to create a sense of togetherness and fostered a sense that we will get through this. Or do you feel some politicians have been nationalistic, lied or ignored the truth because they do not know what to do or perhaps because they lack integrity?

You may feel the scientific advisers have demonstrated leadership based on their knowledge base and ability to communicate, or perhaps not. You may have been inspired by them working on the frontline and perhaps being brave enough to talk about their own experiences and those of their family, or perhaps you consider this a weakness in a leader?

Whatever your thoughts, you need to consider what it is about the person that makes you feel as you do about their leadership and their leadership style and what you can learn from this about your own journey toward being a leader of people.

Activity 1.8 Reflection (p20)

While Karen does a good day-to-day job in making the dialysis unit function, there may be longer-term considerations to take into account. As we saw earlier in the chapter, one of the roles of a leader is operating within the bigger picture. This also resonates with the role of the trained nurse, who has to account not only for the day-to-day running of the dialysis unit but also for the long-term health of the patients. So while it may be all right for the leader to allow someone else to take charge of some of the activities of the team, it is better if they are selective about who takes over what tasks and what they do. The staff in a scenario where it is uncertain who the real leader is will be confused, and may even be slightly angry as they see someone without genuine authority taking control. When you see this in real life it is confusing for patients, staff and students and, in the long term, demoralises and destabilises the team.

Further reading

Barr, J and Dowding, L (2019) *Leadership in Healthcare*. London: Sage.

Especially the first three chapters, which cover much of what is in this chapter in more detail.

Handy, C (1994) *Understanding Organisations* (4th edition). London: Penguin.

The classic text on organisational culture.

Rahman, S and Myers, R (2019) *Courage in Healthcare: A Necessary Virtue or Warning Sign?* London: Sage.

An excellent book examining the need for courage in healthcare practice.

Useful websites

www.businessballs.com

An interesting and quirky leadership and management resources website.

www.kingsfund.org.uk/topics/leadership_and_management/index.html

Perhaps the leading UK healthcare think tank.

http://webarchive.nationalarchives.gov.uk/20150407084231/http://www.midstaffspublicinquiry.com/report

Francis *Report of the Mid Staffordshire NHS Foundation Trust Public Inquiry.*

Chapter 2 · Frameworks for management and leadership

NMC Standards of Proficiency for Registered Nurses

This chapter will address the following platforms and proficiencies:

Platform 1: Being an accountable professional

Registered nurses act in the best interests of people, putting them first and providing nursing care that is person-centred, safe and compassionate. They act professionally at all times and use their knowledge and experience to make evidence-based decisions about care. They communicate effectively, are role models for others, and are accountable for their actions. Registered nurses continually reflect on their practice and keep abreast of new and emerging developments in nursing, health and care.

At the point of registration, the registered nurse will be able to:

1.1 understand and act in accordance with the Code (2018b): Professional standards of practice and behaviour for nurses, midwives and nursing associates, and fulfil all registration requirements.

1.11 communicate effectively using a range of skills and strategies with colleagues and people at all stages of life and with a range of mental, physical, cognitive and behavioural health challenges.

1.14 provide and promote non-discriminatory, person-centred and sensitive care at all times, reflecting on people's values and beliefs, diverse backgrounds, cultural characteristics, language requirements, needs and preferences, taking account of any need for adjustments.

Platform 5: Leading and managing nursing care and working in teams

Registered nurses provide leadership by acting as a role model for best practice in the delivery of nursing care. They are responsible for managing nursing care and are accountable for the appropriate delegation and supervision of care provided by others in the team including

(Continued)

(Continued)

lay carers. They play an active and equal role in the interdisciplinary team, collaborating and communicating effectively with a range of colleagues.

At the point of registration, the registered nurse will be able to:

5.5 safely and effectively lead and manage the nursing care of a group of people, demonstrating appropriate prioritisation, delegation and assignment of care responsibilities to others involved in providing care.

Chapter aims

After reading this chapter, you will be able to:

* identify the features of leadership and management;
* discuss what features of management and leadership are appropriate in nursing;
* relate some management and leadership theories to your own experiences of practice;
* consider which aspects of leadership and management you would like to develop in yourself.

Introduction

The purpose of this chapter is to provide some definition and enable you to understand what it means to be a leader or manager in health and social care. To appreciate leadership and management for nursing fully it is important that any definition of the roles leaders and managers hold includes not just a theoretical explanation of what they do, but also some explanation of how they might be applied in nursing as well as why they are important to practice.

This chapter will advance some of the ideas seen in Chapter 1, where the key characteristics of leaders and managers as might be experienced by student nurses were explored.

Are leadership and management different?

Some commentators on leadership and management regard them to be totally different from each other – a manager is a manager and a leader is a leader. More commonly, and perhaps more correctly, one could say leadership is one of the roles of a manager in health and social care, whereas leadership can be everyone's responsibility depending on their position, the roles they are given and the situations in which they find themselves.

This may seem a difficult idea to grasp, but consider all the people who display leadership qualities, or who undertake leadership roles, in the clinical setting. These people may include individuals who have responsibility for leading a small team, some of whom may be at the same grade. Other leaders may have specific roles in the team, such as a wound care or moving and handling co-ordinator. On occasions people may have to show leadership because of a situation that arises. Such individuals are not perhaps always managers, but they are leaders, even if that leadership is informal, transient and only applies to certain tasks or situations. Informal leadership does not gain much attention in the nursing press but is regarded by some as both important and supportive of teamwork and in the sharing of practice knowledge (Harris and Mayo, 2018).

Managers, on the other hand, are most often defined by their position and job title, e.g. a ward manager, community team manager or outpatients manager. While such individuals are managers, part of their role will include displaying some of the activities of leadership, as described later in the chapter.

Pascale (1990, p65) memorably suggests that: *Managers do things right, while leaders do the right thing.* The proposition here is that managers are bound by and follow policy and procedures, while leaders follow their intuition and understanding of people to get things done. In 1989, Bennis famously explored the comparisons between what he saw as the key features of leadership and listed 12 key differences between managers and leaders:

1. Managers administer; leaders innovate.
2. The manager is a copy; the leader is an original.
3. Managers maintain; leaders develop.
4. Managers focus on systems and structure; leaders focus on people.
5. Managers rely on control; leaders inspire trust.
6. Managers have a short-range view; leaders have a long-range perspective.
7. Managers ask how and when; leaders ask what and why.
8. Managers have their eye always on the bottom line; the leader's eye is on the horizon.
9. Managers imitate; leaders originate.
10. Managers accept the status quo; leaders challenge it.
11. Managers are the classic good soldier; leaders are their own person.
12. Managers do things right; leaders do the right thing.

We can see in these comparisons that managers are regarded as having the interests of the organisation at heart and that they achieve this by following the rules and maintaining the status quo. Perhaps the overwhelming difference is the willingness to try new things, which Bennis regards leaders as having and managers not.

Daft (2001) further expands on Bennis' ideas:

13. Managers plan and budget; leaders create vision and set direction.

14. Managers generally direct and control; leaders allow room for others to grow and change them in the process.

15. Managers create boundaries; leaders reduce them.

16. The manager's relationship with people is based on position power; the leader's relationship and influence are based on personal power.

17. Managers act as bosses; leaders act as coaches, facilitators and servants.

18. Managers exhibit and focus on: emotional distance, expert mind, talking, conformity and insight into the organisation; leaders exhibit and focus on: emotional connectedness, open-mindedness, listening, non-conformity and insight into self.

19. Managers maintain stability; leaders create change.

20. Managers create a culture of efficiency; leaders create a culture of integrity.

What we can see in these definitions is the focus on emotional connections with the team on the part of the leader, and remoteness and control from the manager. What seems clear from these distinctions is some of these qualities will suit some situations at different times, but it is unlikely that one or the other approach will always be right.

It is worth noting again that leadership is also one of the roles of the manager and so the distinctions drawn here may be somewhat artificial. Nurses in the care setting need to demonstrate the qualities of both leaders and managers.

Activity 2.1   Reflection

Think back to some of your experiences in clinical practice and consider the types of leaders and managers you encountered while there. What were the characteristics of the people in charge you admired? Why did you admire these characteristics?

There are some possible answers and thoughts at the end of the chapter.

Considering the differences in the above comparisons and the answers you gave to the activity, you may start to form the opinion that leaders are better than managers in the ways in which they connect with people. You may feel managers perhaps miss the bigger picture and are more remote and removed from the realities of practice. You may also note that some circumstances require management and therefore some of the key skills of management are appropriate to those situations.

In exploring different management and leadership theories in the rest of the chapter, we hope you will start to see, as we have already suggested, that leadership and management styles and activities can co-exist in, and be practised by, the same person. We further hope you will also come to the conclusion that perhaps the art of good leadership and management is knowing what style of supervision to apply in what situation. So being a good manager may also mean being a good leader.

You may find it useful to look back at the answers you gave to some of the activities in Chapter 1 (especially Activities 1.2, 1.5 and 1.6) and consider what role values play in helping to shape leadership and management behaviours. Consideration of the 2018 NMC *Future Nurse: Standards of Proficiency for Registered Nurses*, notably Platform 5 'Leading and managing nursing care and working in teams' (see the start of this chapter), should be at the forefront of your mind as you read the rest of this chapter and engage with the activities and case studies.

While we argue that leadership and management cannot be divorced from each other, it is worth considering theories of management and theories of leadership to see what we can gain from them and when it might be appropriate to adopt one approach or the other in supervising care.

Theories of management

Unlike biochemistry, microbiology and physiology, the study of leadership and management is neither precise nor based on scientific principles. This means there are many theories about what it means to be a leader or a manager, but none of these are proven; they are **theories** (i.e. logical attempts to explain an observation) rather than facts.

The purpose of the theories in the discipline of studying management and leadership is to act as a guide to, or means of explaining, the important tasks and roles of the manager. Interestingly for nursing, a profession increasingly driven by an emphasis on evidence-based practice, little of the work of the manager, especially the health and social care manager, is informed by any meaningful research and it remains theoretical. What this means is that we have theory and observation for guidance, but there is a large amount of scope within these theories for personal interpretation and adjustment to individual management tasks and contexts. There is a large amount of research into leadership and management styles and behaviours from disciplines other than nursing which can be used to inform your thinking, some of which we will refer to in this book.

In part, the lack of meaningful research into the management function is, itself, a product of the diversity of people, staff, managers and settings in which nurse management takes place. The uniqueness of each manager, team, group and organisation, as well as the ever-changing *political, economic, social and technological* climate in which they work, mean it is difficult to produce research-informed strategies for management that have any real, long-lasting meaning. This means that being a manager requires a constant engagement with the people being managed, the organisation and the wider political and social context.

In fact, PEST analyses, using considerations of **p**olitical, **e**conomic, **s**ocial and **t**echnological factors, often alongside **l**egal and **e**nvironmental perspectives (PESTLE), are widely used when trying to make decisions relating to the management of change or organisational development. Scammell (2018), for example, uses a PESTLE analysis to help understand why nurses don't, and why they should, take breaks during the working day.

Activity 2.2   Researching and finding out

Go online and identify the paper by Scammel (the reference is in the further reading at the end of the chapter). Read the paper, then using the same headings from the PESTLE analysis, add your own interpretations as to what is happening in the way of taking breaks where you are currently working or most recently worked.

As this activity is based on your own reflection, there is no specimen answer at the end of the chapter.

What you might see if you were to review this paper is that the interpretations of the different parts of the model are unique to each workplace.

What this implies for theories of management is that they are just that: theories. Theories are ideas about a topic which are supported by some evidence; they are not substantively proven. Even if management theories were proven, they would not necessarily all apply in the same way in every management situation or in every workplace.

Mintzberg's management role theory

Mintzberg (1975) produced one of the most enduring descriptions of the roles of the manager. Mintzberg suggests that if managers are to be effective at what they do, they need to recognise the nature and scope of the work they are undertaking and they must apply their own natural abilities to it. Mintzberg further suggests that the management function is complex and involves an intricate balance of three key roles. The power which the manager possesses arises from a recognition of his or her formal authority and status within the organisation. There are three categories within which the roles of the manager sit, as Mintzberg describes them. These are the *interpersonal*, the *informational* and the *decisional*. Within each of these categories there are a number of roles which together constitute the larger role; that of management.

Interpersonal roles

- Figurehead – the manager performs some more basic functions which may be part of the routine of day-to-day work.

- Leader – including recruitment, staff development and motivating staff.
- Liaison – including communication with people and organisations not directly related to the immediate team.

Informational roles

- Monitor – in this role the manager collects information about the team and the wider environment in which the team works. Some of this information comes from official sources and some from sources such as staff room gossip.
- Disseminator – managers share some of the information they have gathered from formal and informal sources from inside and outside the team with the team. There is a need for discretion here as to what information is shared, with whom and when.
- Spokesperson – essentially information sharing outside of the direct team and organisation.

Decisional roles

- Entrepreneur – the manager seeks opportunities to improve what they do.
- Disturbance handler – the manager must respond to external pressures and make changes that have not come from within the team.
- Resource allocator – as well as managing his or her own time, the manager allocates tasks, equipment and jobs to the team.
- Negotiator – this may mean within the team, with service users, other professions or other agencies. Sometimes this is planned; sometimes it is a response to immediate pressures.

(Adapted from Mintzberg, 1975)

What is apparent from the description of the manager Mintzberg presents is that management requires a fair degree of adaptability. Mintzberg regards the interpersonal elements of the role as being integral to the task of managing and places leadership within the description of the functions of management.

Activity 2.3   Reflection

Consider how the manager in your last/current place of work exercises the various roles of the manager as described by Mintzberg. How does the manager adopting a particular role at a particular time affect you and the rest of the team? Can you identify them moving between roles throughout the day? Perhaps you are, or have been, on your management placement. Are you conscious of the need to do different things at different points in the day? Is the switch between roles something which you consciously do?

As this activity is based on your own reflection, there is no specimen answer at the end of the chapter.

Theories such as Mintzberg's can help to add some clarity to what it is managers do. In Chapter 1, the case study 'The newly qualified nurse' demonstrated that the student (Julius) had little idea about what it was that the ward sister (Deirdre) did all day. Sometimes an understanding of the roles and pressures others work under, in this case the very many roles the manager must practise within a day, allows us to understand better what it is they do and therefore our place in the team.

Contingency theory

Contingency theory refers to the idea that managers must take into account several factors when making management decisions; that is, decisions are situation dependent. Management decisions are therefore seen as being dependent on what is happening, where it is happening and who is involved. This is perhaps best thought of as applying as much to the way in which a decision is made as to the decision that is eventually made. Such an idea fits well within Mintzberg's scheme, where the manager is busy juggling a number of roles in order to fulfil the task of managing dependent on the situation they find themself in as well as the various external influences on this.

Activity 2.4   Reflection

Reflect on the management decisions made on a day-to-day basis in the area in which you are/have most recently been on placement. What are the factors that influence the way in which these decisions are made/communicated and therefore the impact they have on the team? Are these decisions always communicated in an appropriate way? How does the team respond to the manner of the communication?

Since this is based on your own experiences, there is no specimen answer at the end of the chapter.

Contingency theory is similar to the different ways in which you will interact with clients and their relatives according to the nature of the care they are receiving, their age, mental capacity and how well you know them. As a manager, successful action relies on understanding a situation, which in turn relies on good communication. Griffin (2016) makes the useful point that what works as a manager in one situation cannot be generalised to all such situations. As such, managers have to be adaptable to the demands of their various roles as well as the environment they work in and the people they work with.

Systems theory

Systems theory identifies how managing people, resources and care delivery requires the manager to recognise the contribution all these elements make to the effective running of an organisation or team. Systems theorists see the world of work as a set of interdependent subsystems which interconnect to form what is a whole (or holistic) system. Von Bertalanffy (1968), the first and most famous systems theorist, recognised that systems (teams, groups, organisations) are characterised by the interactions of their components (people and their environments) and the unpredictability of those interactions.

What this means for the management of people is that the role each plays within the functioning of a team has to be recognised, supported and directed but with one eye on the bigger picture. When one part of the system fails, then the whole system is affected. It is important, therefore, for the leader or manager to consider the role of each member of the team in achieving the team's goals.

The Hawthorne experiments (see the useful websites at the end of this chapter) provide an interesting insight into how people are motivated at work by the feelings of belonging and of being paid attention to; the so-called **Hawthorne effect**. Essentially the experiments undertaken at the Hawthorne factory involved making both positive and negative changes to people's working conditions and recording the impact this had on productivity. What the experiments demonstrated is that what is done is not as important as the fact that workers are being paid attention to, which alters their behaviour. A similar effect is seen in research, where people react in ways they believe a researcher wants them to because they are under scrutiny (Ellis, 2019a).

Activity 2.5   Research and finding out

Consider the practice area you are most recently familiar with. Make a list of all of the people you have come into contact with who play a role in the day-to-day activity of the area. Do not just list the clinical roles; think about the support, clerical and management services staff who contribute to the running of the area. List what these people do and who is affected by this. Think about the impact on other staff as well as patients, service users or visitors. Consider together what difficulties the rest of the team face when individual members of this wider team are away from work. What does this say about the way in which that system works?

Since this is based on your own experiences, there is no specimen answer at the end of the chapter.

The important message for the manager here is the need to demonstrate to all members of the team that the role they play, however minor it may seem, can have a much wider impact. We saw a wider realisation of this during the 2020 coronavirus pandemic when 'clap for the NHS' became 'clap for key workers' as people at large realised that to function as a society we require not just health and social care, but food, drink, power and, of course, the internet.

Case study: The wrong mop

George is a new ward orderly who is responsible for cleaning Juniper Ward. The ward has three bays. In bay two is a patient with methicillin-resistant *Staphylococcus aureus* (MRSA), who is being nursed in isolation. George mops side room two and then continues to use the same mop to clean the open ward areas. Within a few days there is an outbreak of MRSA on the ward.

This case study reminds us that even the most mundane task can have a significant impact not only on the nursing team, but also the patients that we care for. The nurses on the ward may have been meticulous in their hygiene and infection-control procedures when caring for the MRSA-positive patient, but one component of the system, in this case George, was not and so the system, which includes the ward and the hospital at large, is affected. Of course, there are a few potential explanations for George's lack of understanding about the impact of his actions, which include poor training, poor leadership or perhaps his feeling of not belonging in the ward team.

What should be clear to you in thinking about systems theory is that the team is only as good as the weakest of its members, and everyone has to play a part in achieving a task, no matter how mundane that task is. One of the lessons from this for the nurse on their journey to leadership and management is to consider, and pay attention to, all the members of the team, not just the 'most important' or the most senior.

Workload management

Within the role of the manager there are several tasks which need to be undertaken. Some of these tasks reflect on the roles identified in the model by Mintzberg; others are more singular and are worthy of some discussion here.

The role of the manager in co-ordinating the work of a team was alluded to in Chapter 1, especially in the case study 'The newly qualified nurse'. The management of workload is perhaps one of the key skills for the new or aspiring nurse manager who needs to satisfy his or her own developmental and work–life balance needs; the needs of the team members; the needs of the organisation; and the needs of the people who use the service.

To achieve this balance the nurse manager must learn and consolidate a number of skills and, while this is not an exhaustive list, some of these skills are discussed here:

- Learn to say 'no'! The need to prioritise workloads as a manager is very real (Chunta, 2020). Taking on more than you or the team can manage will mean that no one is satisfied.

- Learn to delegate. People are the greatest resource for the nurse leader and manager. Knowing your team, what they are capable of and what individuals enjoy doing means that you can delegate tasks and everyone benefits (Ellis, 2015).
- Manage your time with the team (Kruse, 2019). When you have a pressing task to attend to, an open-door policy (which allows anyone in at any time for any reason) means you cannot concentrate on what is in front of you and so are unable to finish anything, so it is a good idea to close the metaphorical door on some occasions. Clearly this is not always appropriate; emergency situations may require immediate attention and shutting yourself away during a crisis is not helpful.
- Learn to go home. If your job cannot be done in the time allotted to it, you have too much work. A tired nurse manager is likely to make mistakes and burn out (Kelly et al., 2019). This is no good to anyone. Failure to achieve everything in the allotted time may also indicate the need to become more organised, delegate more effectively and manage time more wisely.

By managing their time through prioritising, saying no and sensible delegation, managers can achieve their goals and develop team members at the same time. In Chapter 6 we discuss burnout. Some burnout can be attributed to not taking care of oneself as a manager, working too many hours and not having a good work–life balance. While the perfect work–life balance for most remains a unobtainable dream, leaders do need to consider the impact of overworking not only on themselves but also on the message it sends to the wider team.

Of the roles of the nurse manager, drawing up the roster is one which can often lead to disagreement and create disharmony in the team (as we will see in the case study 'The rota' in Chapter 5). For the manager who is concerned with doing things right, there are a few simple rules to follow in undertaking this task and which contribute to successful workload.

There is a need to be open and honest about the process: people have no need to speculate and gossip about what they can see. An open process will involve observing two important principles: being fair and being consistent. *The Code* (NMC, 2018b, p18) requires the nurse to show integrity, honesty and act in ways so that you are *aware at all times of how your behaviour can affect and influence the behaviour of other people.* Clearly, as well as being transparent in the process of work allocation, it is important for the manager to allocate staff so that there are appropriate levels (the skill mix) and numbers of staff on duty at any one time.

The sorts of principles associated with moral management are also the sorts of principles associated with moral and ethical nursing practice. Fairness dictates that all staff are given equal opportunity to request days off and consistency that these are all considered according to the same criteria. Whatever tasks the manager faces, be this acting as a spokesperson or as a role model (see the NMC's Platform 5, at the start of the chapter), there is a need to demonstrate moral and ethical awareness. Managers who are unable to demonstrate moral activity in their day-to-day management practice cannot reasonably require the same from their team. Moral and professional conduct is perhaps the cornerstone of good nursing and management practice.

Resilience and management

One of the features of modern nursing management is the need to be resilient. Resilience is the ability to cope with, and even thrive despite the stresses and challenges that being a twenty-first-century nurse manager throw up. In Chapter 9, we will discuss strategies for developing confidence as a leader or manager and how this will enable you to make the transitions from student to qualified nurse and nurse leader.

The most important strategy in being resilient is your own ability to make sense of what is happening in the world around you. In part, this ability comes from a strong understanding and belief in your core values (as discussed in Chapter 1). A positive attitude to reflecting on and learning from changes and challenges (see 'The learning organisation' in Chapter 6) is a core element of being a good nurse and, later, a good nurse manager. This understanding is exercised and communicated using emotional intelligence (as described in Chapter 5, as well as later in this chapter) in which the leader recognises and responds to his or her own, and other people's, emotional responses to a situation rather than dealing with it on a purely cognitive (thinking) level.

Being positive and using new situations as opportunities to learn means you will develop problem-solving abilities. The ability to solve problems means that you are in control, not only of the situation, but also of yourself.

Ellis and Abbott (2017, p289) caution:

> *Resilience requires the manager to understand themself and the things which affect them because in this way the manager can manage their response to situations. It is important here to understand that the manager who develops a thick skin does not learn, does not see what is going on around them and will lack the emotional intelligence and empathy to deal with the people elements of the role.*

So resilience is not about hiding away and disengaging from one's emotional responses to situations; it is about learning what your responses are and then learning how to manage them.

Activity 2.6   Reflection

Consider how reflection on critical incidents throughout your training as a nurse has enabled you to make sense of some aspects of nursing practice. What strategies did you find helpful during this process – perhaps discussion with peers, tutors, practice supervisors or managers, reading articles, textbooks or attending lectures? How did this process help you to develop? What was it about reflection that enabled you to cope in untoward circumstances? Compare how you cope with untoward incidents now with how you coped before you started to train as a nurse; what are the differences? How might these strategies translate to the need for resilience as a leader or manager?

There are some possible answers and thoughts at the end of the chapter.

Your reflections on this activity will have led you to the conclusion that being prepared emotionally and intellectually is one of the key strategies for surviving as a student, as a nurse and, in the long term, as a manager. As with all aspects of leadership and management, understanding your own responses to a situation will mean you are better prepared for, and more understanding of, the emotional responses of others. That is one of the fundamental requirements of effective people management.

Theories of leadership

Leadership can be regarded as one facet of the management role or as an entity in itself. It is a people-focused activity that requires engagement with a team – the followers. The King's Fund (2015) identify how leaders in healthcare are consistent in motivating others while promoting continued staff development in order to improve patient outcomes.

Remember, being a leader can arise out of an individual's position within an organisation, or their natural ability to inspire other people to follow them. There are several approaches to leadership, some of which take account of the nature of the interaction between the leader and followers and others which take a more comprehensive view of the nature of leadership and the tasks of the leader as well as the interpersonal aspect of the role.

Every leader has their own definition and understanding of what leadership is about, many share similarities and all make reference to some broadly similar key points. Grint et al. (2017) point out that there are five elements to defining leadership:

1. *Leadership as a Person: the concept of WHO someone is making them a leader*
2. *Leadership as a Result: it is WHAT the person can accomplish which makes them a leader*
3. *Leadership as a Position: refers to WHERE the leadership takes place and the job they are in which defines them as a leader*
4. *Leadership as a Purpose: understanding WHY someone chose to lead defines their approach to leadership*
5. *Leadership as a Process: HOW a person leads making them a leader.*

What is interesting about this idea is that it is equally possible to define leadership as a task and situational as it is as person and positional; this reinforces how difficult it is to come to one single definition of leadership.

Transactional leadership

Transactional leadership is leadership at its most basic. As the name implies, there is a transaction taking place. The followers do what the leader asks of them in return for a reward, at its most basic a salary or perhaps praise or recognition. The role of the leader in this model is to state what needs to be done and who will do it, allow them to get the job done and provide the reward.

This approach to leadership is very much focused on getting a task done, rather than on the people undertaking the task. It is easy to imagine how this approach to leadership may be appealing in an emergency. In nursing, it does hark back to the days of task allocation, when patient care was perhaps less holistic.

Relating the theory to good leadership practice, the leader who understands and communicates effectively with the team will gain the respect and trust of that team and for the team the reward for getting the job done will come from the sense of shared purpose and belonging that co-operative working brings. That said, at its most basic, transactional leadership is not very engaging for the leader or the team members and does not recognise, or promote, innovation and professional practice.

Transformational leadership

Transformational leadership is about having a vision (a view of how things should or could be) and being able to communicate this vision effectively. The vision of how things should be may come from leaders themselves, from their managers or following discussion within a group or team. What is important about transformational leaders is that they believe, and are seen to believe, the vision.

For transformational leadership to work, there are some assumptions which need to be made and need to be true. First, people will follow a leader who can inspire them; second, a passionate leader with vision can get things done; and third, getting things done is a matter of instilling energy and enthusiasm into a group.

Transformational leadership requires there to be a relationship of trust between the leader and their followers. This trust means the followers will do whatever it is that the leader envisions for them. As in all relationships, the best way to generate trust is to show people you care about them and be consistent in your approach to achieving the management task (Scholtes, 1998 – see p45).

Transformational leaders succeed in what they do by having faith, not only in what they want to achieve and what they do, but also by generating and displaying trust in those they work with. Clearly one of the central focuses of the transformational leader is change, or perhaps more accurately, transformational progress. Transformational leaders who are successful in sharing their vision with their team will doubtless be able to lead their team through change more successfully than leaders who do not have the full support of the team.

It is worth considering whether transformational leadership is suited to health and social care and, more specifically, nursing. The simple answer is that the most successful nurse leaders will retain a vision of how things should be in terms of high-quality and successful patient care provision. The shared values of care and compassion are the key to generating the trust which transformational leaders need to improve (transform) care provision.

Of course, having the faith and trust of the team is not, in itself, enough to make a person a transformational leader. There is also a real need for a vision that is correct and workable as well as inspiring. If we can agree that all improvement is a change, but not all change is an improvement, we can see that enthusiasm and vision without some foundation in reality are perhaps not all that helpful. Trust is generated when followers believe both that a leader cares about them as individuals and that the same leader can deliver whatever it is they say they will deliver. Liking someone as an individual and trusting that person as a leader are not the same thing.

Activity 2.7   Reflection

Think about an occasion when you have met a practice supervisor or lecturer who you have liked because they were inspirational. Now think about whether they delivered what you expected. Did you learn what you thought you would learn? What was the difference between successful learning and less successful learning? Is a good relationship as important for learning as the content of the learning?

There are some possible answers and thoughts at the end of the chapter.

What this reflection shows is that there is more than one dimension to being an effective leader of people. Being nice is not enough; there is a need for some substance to underpin activity. The best leaders both inspire confidence in their ability and demonstrate they care about the team as well as the work which needs to be done.

Bass and Riggio (2014) suggest four essential components of effective transformational leadership. First, leaders must provide intellectual stimulation, challenging the way things are and encouraging creativity among the team. Second, they must demonstrate individualised consideration and, by using good communication skills, make followers feel able to share ideas and gain direct recognition for their unique contributions. Third, they need to demonstrate inspirational motivation which enables followers to experience the same passion and motivation as the leader to meet the team goals.

Fourth, they need to have idealised influence; that is, they must act as a role model who followers wish to emulate while taking on the values of the leader.

Reflecting on the nature of the leaders we respect and trust, the sorts of people we choose as role models, we can see they have many of the characteristics which suggest they are exercising values which are central to nursing. The requirements of a transformational leader closely reflect what Jane Cummings, the Chief Nurse for NHS England, in 2012 coined as the 6 Cs (see the useful websites at the end of the chapter).

1. *care*
2. *compassion*
3. *competence*
4. *communication*
5. *courage*
6. *commitment.*

Transformational leaders who have the ability to exercise, and be seen to exercise, these essential values in their dealings with colleagues and service users can expect others to see these as a template for how they ought to act. One of the core learning points for anyone moving into a leadership or management position in the caring professions is not to put aside the qualities and values they worked to while in clinical practice (as embodied in the 6 Cs), since their continued exercise reflects strongly on who we are. Putting aside our values, as we discussed in the scenario about Julius and Deirdre, can lead to dire consequences for all concerned.

Activity 2.8   Research and finding out

Go online and find some more information about transformational leadership. Identify what various sites say are the qualities of a transformational leader. What examples can you find of transformational leaders in history, or more recently during the worldwide COVID-19 pandemic? What, if any, attributes do you share with these great transformational leaders? Which might you be able to cultivate for yourself in the coming years?

Since this is based on your own experiences, there is no specimen answer at the end of the chapter.

Adair's action-centred leadership

Adair (2010) describes leadership as being made up of three interlocking and interdependent activities (often portrayed as interconnected circles (see Figure 2.1)) which leaders must pay attention to in their role: the task, the team and the individual. The role of the leader is to achieve the task (in nursing, this may be the provision of good-quality care) through building and developing the team while developing the individuals who make up the team.

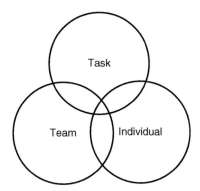

Figure 2.1   Action-centred leadership

Source: Adapted from Adair (2010).

The functions of the leader, as described by Adair (2010), which enable them to achieve the task are: defining the task, planning how the task will be achieved, briefing the team and controlling the process. To achieve the task the leader also needs to pay attention to the human elements of what they are doing through evaluating, motivating, organising and providing an example to both the team and the individuals in it. The elements of the various activities include:

Task

- Organising duties
- Focusing on goals
- Controlling quality
- Checking performance
- Reviewing progress.

Team

- Building and maintaining morale
- Maintaining communication
- Setting standards
- Supporting the team.

Individual

- Praise and recognition
- Developing and training
- Meeting human needs.

Ignoring or underemphasising any one of these areas of activity will mean the leader is not doing what the team, individual or task require. Overemphasis on any one element of these three leadership activities will lead to imbalances in the ways in which work is done. Leaders need to learn to balance all three activity areas as a rule, increasing their attention in any one area for short periods as required. So, for instance, if there are problems with the team the effort put into this needs to increase, but – and this is important – this should not mean the leader neglects the task or the individuals within the team as a result.

The servant leader

Many classic models of leadership identify the leader as the individual out in front with the followers coming along behind. Some modern theories of leadership take a different view of the role of leaders, who have a more interdependent relationship with their team (Ellis, 2021a). The role of the leader in this view is that of a leader who also has the ability to follow. This idea of the 'servant leader' is described as an individual who wants to serve first and to whom the decision to lead comes later. Servant leaders seek leadership as a means of expanding their ability to serve. In some respects, there is a relationship between this and systems theory, in that the servant leader appreciates their role as leader is to co-ordinate the activity of the system (the team/organisation) to achieve the shared (system) goals of the team or organisation.

Throughout history there have been several individuals who can be said to have been servant leaders. Well-known examples include the Dalai Lama, Mahatma Gandhi and Mother Teresa. These individuals, whose motivation lies in serving others, have managed to expand their ability to do so by taking on leadership roles. While it can be argued that each was motivated by religion or political change, they share the value of care for other people, which is a value common to many healthcare managers and leaders.

Activity 2.9   Reflection

Consider the nursing leaders who have left an impression on you. Do not worry whether that impression was positive or negative, or about the grade or seniority of the leader. Identify why that leader left an impression on you. Consider issues like their ability to get things done, their relationships with others (both individually and with the team) and what values they displayed (or failed to display). Consider how that person made you feel and why. Think then about what the attributes of a good leader might be, given your personal experiences.

Reflecting on what you have identified as the strengths and weaknesses of the leaders you have worked with, now consider your own development as a leader and how you will behave around others.

As this is based on your own thoughts and reflections, there is no specimen answer at the end of the chapter.

We can see from this reflection that servant leadership could be a natural progression for nurses who start their career in positions where they deliver patient care. This model of leadership allows there to be some consistency in who they are and what they do as their career progresses. They demonstrate connectedness with their team members both as a group and as individuals, while always knowing what it is they want to achieve.

Being a servant leader should not be used as justification for leaders and managers to continue to deliver nursing care most of the time while neglecting the role which they are paid to perform. While we have highlighted the person-centred nature of health and social care, this does not mean leaders or managers have to deliver face-to-face patient care. What it does mean is that they need to support their staff to do so by leading by example, providing environments conducive to learning and improving care (see Chapter 8) and by creating and supporting policies which underpin person-centred care.

The NHS Leadership Model

Partly in response to the Francis report (2013) and partly to update an old leadership framework, the NHS Leadership Academy launched the new Healthcare Leadership Model in 2013. The emphasis of the model is on personal qualities and behaviours. The authors argue:

> *The way that we manage ourselves is a central part of being an effective leader. It is vital to recognise that personal qualities like self-awareness, self-confidence, self-control, self-knowledge, personal reflection, resilience and determination are the foundation of how we behave. Being aware of your strengths and limitations in these areas will have a direct effect on how you behave and interact with others, and they with you.*

(NHS Leadership Academy, 2013)

The argument continues to highlight how the behaviours of the leader set the culture of the workplace and, subsequently, the manner in which patient care is delivered. In their view, workplace culture is partly a product of the behaviours and dispositions of the leader. Ideas regarding personal qualities are not explicit in the model but are a core theme throughout. Being able to lead with reference to personal qualities and exhibited behaviours requires self-awareness and emotional intelligence. The model is divided into nine interdependent and interlocked dimensions.

The nine dimensions of the Healthcare Leadership Model

1. Inspiring shared purpose
2. Leading with care
3. Evaluating information

4. Connecting our service

5. Sharing the vision

6. Engaging the team

7. Holding to account

8. Developing capability

9. Influencing for results

Activity 2.10   Research and finding out

Go online and find the NHS Healthcare Leadership Model (use the web address given at the end of this chapter). Read each of the descriptors for each dimension and reflect on how they describe what each dimension is, is not and why it is important. Look at the four-part scale which describes a person's engagement with each dimension of the model (essential, proficient, strong and exemplary) and consider which description best fits you. You might also consider how the manager or leader in your most recent placement might score against the different dimensions.

Since this is based on your own experiences, there is no specimen answer at the end of the chapter.

The role of emotional intelligence

The concept of emotional intelligence has gained an increasing following over recent years. Emotional intelligence in relation to leadership and management refers to the ability of leaders or managers to understand the role that their emotions play in their decision-making and the ability to recognise the emotions of the individuals within the team and how this affects the work they do (Goleman, 1996).

Recognising the influence of emotions on decision-making means leaders and managers may be in a better position to understand what motivates and what constrains staff in their work. Leaders and managers who have well-developed emotional intelligence are said to be better at communicating with their team and therefore at achieving better outcomes.

Goleman (1998, p317) defines emotional intelligence as the capacity for recognising our own feelings and those of others, for motivating ourselves, and for managing emotions well in ourselves and in our relationships. He further states that emotional intelligence is a learned capability. Goleman's emotional intelligence framework comprises five elements: self-awareness, motivation, self-regulation, empathy and social skills. It is probably fair to comment that emotional intelligence is one dimension of what it is to be a good nurse and that this learned skill translates well into leadership and management roles.

It follows from this, however, that people who rely heavily on their emotions to guide their actions will tend to base their decisions on their emotional responses to a situation rather than on more objective empirical evidence. Raghubir (2018) suggests, however, that emotional intelligence should be used to gain an understanding of the emotional needs and concerns of the patient and it is this understanding, and not the emotions and values of the nurse, which should guide clinical decision-making. That said, the failure of leaders and managers to understand the role of their own emotions and those of their staff in shaping decision-making and behaviours at work will mean that important issues are overlooked which may affect patient care.

Case study: The grieving staff nurse

Blossom had always been a self-confident and able staff nurse. She was friendly with staff and patients, but on the whole tended to keep very much to herself. Blossom had seemed a little withdrawn in recent weeks but had said nothing to anyone until one day she went into an unexplained rage. Blossom shouted at the students and her fellow staff nurses and was rude and abrasive toward patients and visitors. Kathy, a fellow staff nurse, decided she should take control of the situation and took Blossom to one side. Once in the ward office Blossom started to cry. She confided to Kathy that her father had died some weeks previously and she was finding it hard to cope.

There are two interesting elements to this case study: first, Blossom had not shared her grief with anyone and did not know how to deal with it herself; second, no one on the ward team had picked up on her distress. On two levels, then, emotional intelligence was seen to be lacking: in Blossom recognising the effects of grief on her behaviour, and in her colleagues recognising that Blossom was grieving. For emotional intelligence to work for leaders or managers of people, those managers need to have a relationship with their individual staff members, otherwise changes in their emotional status will go unnoticed.

Chapter 5 looks at emotional intelligence in the context of conflict management.

Gaining support

What we have seen in this chapter is that one of the key roles of leaders or managers in nursing is working with and through their team. In order to achieve this, nurse managers and leaders need the support of their team. How this support is gained and maintained is through a mixture of good communication, good interpersonal skills and developing a sense of achievement. The team will support a leader that they trust.

Scholtes (1998) identifies trust as arising out of the feeling that leaders or managers both care for their staff and are capable of doing the job (Figure 2.2).

The model presented in Figure 2.2 demonstrates to novice leaders or managers the importance not only of getting the technical, procedural and policy elements of their role right, but also the need to take their team with them. This returns us to one of the key themes of the chapter – that to be a successful nurse manager there is a clear need not only to know what you are doing, but also to nurture and develop your staff and team while you are doing it – good management and good leadership. Leaders and managers who fail to regard the well-being of their staff as their role will ultimately fail to deliver the best care.

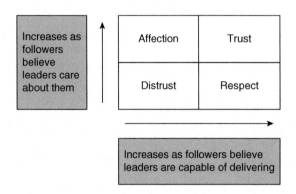

Figure 2.2   Trust, respect and affection

Source: Adapted from Scholtes (1998).

Chapter summary

This chapter has introduced some of the different theories of management and leadership as well as some of the ways of acting that contribute to their success. We have seen that leadership and management, while often viewed as separate entities, can co-exist in the same individual, and that when they do they can add to the success of the manager.

The chapter has identified that some of the key values of nursing translate well into good nurse leadership, that managers or leaders need both resilience and the ability to influence people if they are to be successful. The need for resilience clearly comes from the requirement for managers and leaders to manage what can be difficult situations, and part of the toolkit of successful leadership and management in terms of resilience is the ability to connect with people on the human level and thereby influence what they do and how they do it.

For nurses, who enter the profession to care for others, maintaining the focus on care as a fundamental part of developing as a leader and manager both sets a good role model to the team and helps to develop trust. Developing trust means that nurse leaders or managers can effectively lead their team in the delivery of high-quality nursing care.

Activities: Brief outline answers

Activity 2.1 Reflection (p28)

You may remember meeting staff who were able to let you know what they were doing and why you should do things in the way they wanted. Others may have told you to do things 'because that is how things are done here'. The first example is of leadership, as the senior lets you see why and how you should behave in a certain way. The second example is more managerial in telling you what to do because this is policy. The best senior staff will be able to swap between being a leader and manager according to the situation and this change will appear appropriate; for example, during an emergency it may be best to be told what to do rather than why, with explanation happening after the event.

Activity 2.6 Reflection (p36)

Using reflection as a tool and utilising the experience and understanding of others allow us to see situations in a context. Understanding the context of a situation and why things happen as they do enables us to make sense of them, and cope emotionally with things which might otherwise prove too difficult. Part of the reflection process is planning how we will meet challenges in the future, namely action planning, which is how we become prepared. When we are prepared, we know not only how we will feel, but also how we will act and, more importantly, why. This means that when we meet similar situations in the future they will be less daunting. That is resilience.

Activity 2.7 Reflection (p39)

How you feel about an individual that you have to work with or follow is often affected by whether you like him or her as a person and whether you feel they care about you as an individual. This is certainly an important first step in any relationship. When these same people deliver what they promise, when you learn from them what they said you would learn, it generates a feeling of great trust and gratitude. When an individual that you like is unable to deliver what they promised, you may not stop liking that person, but you question whether your trust in them is well placed and you will think twice before following whatever they say in the future.

Further reading

Adair, J (2010) *Develop Your Leadership Skills*. London: Kogan Page.

A really short and useful introduction to leadership as Adair sees it.

Barr, J and **Dowding, L** (2019) *Leadership in Healthcare* (4th edition). London: Sage.

Especially the first four chapters, which set the scene for leadership and management.

Gopee, N and **Galloway, J** (2017) *Leadership and Management in Healthcare* (3rd edition). London: Sage.

Especially chapter two on the duty care manager and management theories.

Scammell, J (2018) Do you take your breaks? How to influence change in the workplace. *British Journal of Nursing*, 27(9): 514 doi: 10.12968/bjon.2018.27.9.514.

An easy to identify use of the PESTLE analysis.

Useful websites

www.kingsfund.org.uk/Leadership

The King's Fund – a good leadership and management resource website.

www.bbc.co.uk/programmes/b00lv0wx

A podcast and explanation of the Hawthorne effect, which is worth listening to.

www.leadershipacademy.nhs.uk/resources/healthcare-leadership-model

Look here to do the Healthcare Leadership Model activities alluded to in the text.

www.england.nhs.uk/6cs/wp-content/uploads/sites/25/2015/03/introducing-the-6cs.pdf

Explanation of the 6 Cs in the form of a presentation.

Chapter 3 · Teams and teamwork

Chapter aims

After reading this chapter, you will be able to:

- understand team roles and dynamics and how these affect decision-making and team working;
- explore methods to evaluate effective team working;
- consider the skills needed to lead teams, meetings and working groups;
- explore the usefulness of interagency and interdisciplinary team working in healthcare delivery.

Introduction

This chapter will begin by reflecting on your experiences of working in teams and then will progress to exploring how you can develop the skills to manage and lead a team. Nurses, like all professional groups, learn through education and experience to make autonomous and independent professional decisions when managing patient care. At the same time, in health and social care environments, there is an expectation for nurses to:

- work within teams of other nurses (e.g. in wards or units);
- work with interdisciplinary teams (e.g. specialist teams, including doctors and other allied healthcare professionals);
- manage and direct teams with specific specialties (e.g. infection control);
- lead teams to introduce new ways of working or maintain high standards of care (e.g. audit, clinical improvement and task and finish groups).

The chapter will examine how teams work and how to evaluate the effectiveness of teams. The different roles team members assume are covered next, as are skills for improving team working, dealing with difficulties involving team members and team communication. In this section we also explore some of the theoretical positions, based upon social psychology, which have helped to explain team members' behaviour. The practicalities of leading team meetings are described and, finally, the role of interdisciplinary team working is discussed.

How teams work

Understanding group dynamics is the starting point for recognising how teams are formed and how they work at their most productive. It may seem that some groups work well together as if by magic but, in reality, it often needs a deeper understanding of the nature of individuals and how they interact in groups, to create and sustain useful teams.

Tuckman (1965) is the most often quoted commentator on how groups come together. In Tuckman's view there are five stages to the creation of groups:

1. *Forming: the group comes together and the task identified and allocated. At this stage the group may not know each other, but may share similar goals.*

2. *Storming: the group starts to explore how to tackle the allocated task. Relationships in the group start to build, although in some cases this never happens and the group gets stuck in this phase.*

3. *Norming: the group has moved through storming and working practices start to emerge.*

4. *Performing: not all groups get to this stage. Groups that get to this stage are highly independent and motivated.*

5. *Adjourning: once the project, the reason for forming the group, is completed, the group has no further reason to meet and will adjourn.*

Activity 3.1   Reflection

Think of the current, or last, team or group in which you worked. Think about the key activities of the group or team and make a list of what they did together. Would you describe the experience as one where individuals came together for personally focused but unifying relationships, such as those found in families, religious groups, political affiliations or students studying the same module? Or did the experience involve a number of persons associated together in specific work, activity or task, perhaps working toward a common goal or with a set of particular aim and objectives?

If it was the former, this would be described as a group activity. If it was the latter, it would be described as a team. A well-functioning team has:

- defined objectives;
- positive relationships;
- a supportive environment;
- a spirit of co-operation and collaboration.

Since this is based on your own thoughts and reflections, there is no specimen answer at the end of the chapter.

In summary, a team is created from a number of people who are all organised to function co-operatively as a unit. By contrast, a group is deemed to be a number of people sharing something in common, such as an interest, belief or political aim. In common with wider organisations, teams exist to get a job of work done (Tamunomiebi and Uhuru, 2018) and, like organisations, the purpose of teams is to get the job done efficiently and effectively.

Activity 3.2 Critical thinking

Think about a time when you were involved in working in a team. This could be the experience you thought of in Activity 3.1 if it fits the definition of a team. Write down the main aim or purpose of the team. Find out if the team/organisation has a values and vision statement, an area philosophy or statement of purpose (e.g. a ward philosophy). Consider the behaviours in the team that reflect these stated values and, therefore, if the statement contributed to the success or otherwise of the team.

There are some possible answers and thoughts at the end of the chapter.

It is often said that a team as a whole is more effective than the sum of its parts (Lingard et al., 2017); that is to say, a team can get more done and get it done more effectively than the same number of individuals undertaking the task alone or in an unco-ordinated fashion. What do you think it is about teams that makes them more efficient and effective?

Team effectiveness

When a team works well together, this is reflected in the culture and atmosphere of the workplace. This is noticeable in several different ways, for example when team members:

- have a shared understanding of team goals and tasks;
- are willing to listen to each other;
- feel comfortable discussing their work with each other;
- handle disagreements positively and openly;
- demonstrate the team values in their day-to-day work activities;
- give and receive feedback with respect for each other's feelings.

Activity 3.3 Reflection

Compare the list of attributes of an effective team, listed above, to the list of problems which Francis (2013) identified in the *Report of the Mid Staffordshire NHS Foundation Trust Public Inquiry*, discussed in Chapter 1.

Reflect on what this means for the role of values in the creation and effective working of teams.

There are some possible answers and thoughts at the end of the chapter.

In contrast to effective teams, an ineffective team can be dominated by a few members with strong views, opinions and characters. This can mean other members feel isolated from the main purpose of the team, which in turn can lead to feelings such as disenfranchisement, boredom and a lack of engagement and commitment.

An overuse of rules and regulations can lead to a stifling of informal relationship building, a process necessary to achieve team harmony and a supportive atmosphere. For example, each team will have a set of norms to guide it on how each person should be addressed – whether by organisational title and family name, or by first name. Another example might occur when a team has devised a specific method of dealing with patients' personal effects that fits fundamentally with the principles of the organisation's policy, but which has been tested and proven to be less than practical given the nature of the unit – such as an emergency care unit – where people are constantly being moved around. On the other hand, a leader needs to know which institutional or legal regulations must be followed for patient, and organisational, safety to be maintained. Individual team members should also be aware of their own professional responsibilities and accountability, guided by professional codes of conduct such as the NMC *Code* (NMC, 2018b). Acknowledging individuals' responsibility also reinforces a sense of professional autonomy that can contribute positively to (or indeed detract from) team working.

Conflicts and disagreements are uncomfortable situations to deal with in a team. However, if not dealt with, these situations can lead to team members avoiding each other and suppressing negative feelings. This, in turn, can lead to resentment and frustration. So, it is important to look at disagreements as opportunities for improving team relationships, by talking through differences and discussing alternative ways of working together. Team leaders can facilitate these discussions or they can be just between the individuals, provided ground rules are established and resolution of the differences is made a focal objective. A helpful team activity for dealing with differences is for the team to develop a team code of co-operation. (See the useful websites section at the end of this chapter, as well as Chapter 5, for further information on dealing with conflict.) As a rule, people who appear difficult within a team need to be listened to, because it is often the sceptic who helps the team avoid making mistakes, while the overly eager team member might just know something which will be useful to the team if they take the time to listen.

In some situations where issues arise between team members, the manager may need to mediate. Ideally in a team of adults working together, team members who have issues with each other will address these themselves first and managers should encourage staff to do so before being drawn into inter-staff issues. That said, where team effectiveness is impacted by issues between staff members it is the role of the manager to make sure these are sorted out.

Giving feedback on performance to team members (whether you are a leader or from one co-worker to another) is an activity that must happen as and when the need arises, as well as at set points throughout the year, such as at supervision or appraisals. Effective feedback can enhance individual performance and improve the outcomes for the team – which means for patients. Done badly, or too infrequently, feedback can come across as negative and fail in its purpose, which is to improve performance. Chapter 4 looks more closely at working with individuals within teams, and Chapter 6 considers the benefits of coaching and practice assessment.

Negative or destructive criticism that is personal and hurtful has the potential to create discordant relationships that lead to resentment which can, in turn, lead to a lack of co-operation between individuals. While poor performance might warrant negative feedback, the interaction needs to be positive and concentrate on the opportunities for individual and team development. One way for a team to learn to work with constructive feedback is to practise, or role play, in a simulated situation, by giving feedback to one another. This allows team members to experience what it feels like, and to generate phrases that are acceptable to convey feedback to one another in a respectful manner, as shown in Table 3.1.

Attribute	Effective team	Ineffective team
Goals	Are understood and supported	Unclear tasks and objectives
Contributions	Whole team involved and make pertinent contribution	A few members dominate, others are minimised
Environment	Informal and relaxed	Bored and tense
Leadership	Shared and moves with need for expertise	Autocratic
Assignments	Clear allocations which are accepted	Unclear about who is doing what
Listening	Attentive listening with everyone heard	No one listening, ideas ignored or overridden
Conflict	Comfortable with disagreement	Disagreements ignored; minority disenfranchised
Decision-making	By consensus	Actions or voting before issues thought through
Self-evaluation	Ongoing evaluation	Not discussed

Table 3.1 Summary of effective and ineffective team characteristics

Source: Adapted from Yoder-Wise (2019), p339.

Team dynamics and processes

The way team members engage with each other and the factors that affect team functioning are crucial aspects of effective team working. It is customary for there to be a designated team leader who will guide the team, set the tone for how a team will work together and generate performance targets or goals. There are occasions, however, when a team will be self-directed and led jointly by members who have similar status or responsibilities, such as when a multidisciplinary team works together to achieve a common goal.

Norms

Most teams develop norms, which are the informal rules of behaviour shared and enforced by team members. These norms are developed by the team as a form of self-regulation to enable stable team functioning and survival. Norms are often linked to expected contributions from individuals who fulfil specific roles. For example, a student nurse's contribution to the team will be bounded by their being supernumerary, what they are allowed to do, and by how far they are into their training. A healthcare assistant will have specific roles within the team, which relate to their experience and qualifications, as will the qualified nurse who will often be leading others in the team. In established, functional teams, each member will understand their role and support each other with the agreed activities within the well-understood parameters of their responsibilities and capabilities.

However, these parameters may vary from team to team and ward to ward, depending on local policy, the nature of the work, or the experience and qualifications of the team members. Trying to adapt to these different parameters can sometimes lead to misunderstandings because of the variations between teams, and student nurses or new team members will need to find out the norms of any group by discussion and reference to unit protocols. Examples of norms may include when breaks are taken, how shifts are negotiated, how to prevent embarrassment by being loyal to the team, and how collectively held values or principles are best expressed. The assimilation and adaption into a team is a further example of socialisation, which we discussed in Chapter 1.

Roles

A role is an expected set of behaviours that are characteristic of a specific function in the team. Individuals may have an inherent tendency to perform a role, such as a nurturing role; alternatively, roles may be informally ascribed by the group or formally designated by the leader. Benne and Sheats (1948, p43) famously suggested roles can be divided into either task roles or nurturing roles, and these are set out in Tables 3.2 and 3.3, respectively.

Task roles keep the team focused on their objectives or functions, whereas nurturing roles are facilitative or concerned with meeting interpersonal needs. Team members may adopt more than one role. A team leader may wish to accentuate one role in place of another to improve team functioning or, alternatively, to suppress a role that becomes over-emphasised. Learning when to do this and what benefits accrue from it is one of the skills of good leadership. It is in doing this that the team leader assumes the

Initiator	Redefines problems and offers solutions, clarifies objectives
Contributor	Suggests agenda items and maintains time limits
Information seeker	Pursues descriptive baseline information for the team's work
Information giver	Expands information given by sharing experiences and making inferences
Opinion seeker	Explores viewpoints that clarify or reflect the values of other members' suggestions
Opinion giver	Conveys to group members what their essential values should be
Elaborator	Predicts outcomes and provides illustrations or expands suggestions, clarifying how they could work
Co-ordinator	Links ideas or suggestions offered by others
Orienter	Summarises the group's discussions and actions
Evaluator critic	Appraises the quantity and quality of the team's accomplishments against set standards
Energiser	Motivates the group to accomplish, qualitatively and quantitatively, the team's goals
Procedural technician	Supports team activity by arranging the environment and providing necessary equipment
Recorder	Documents the team's progress, actions and achievements

Table 3.2   Task roles

Encourager	Compliments members for their opinions and contributions to the team
Harmoniser	Relieves tensions and conflicts
Compromiser	Sets aside own position or views to maintain team harmony
Gate keeper	Stimulates discussion to enable all team members to communicate and participate, without allowing any one member to dominate
Group observer	Notices team processes and dynamics and informs the team of them
Follower	Passively attends meetings, listens to discussions and accepts the team's decisions

Table 3.3   Nurturing roles

role of a conductor of an orchestra, utilising the different talents of the team, at different times, to achieve a successful performance.

Meredith Belbin (2010) continues to be one of the major contributors to team role theory. Based on research into dysfunctional teams in the 1970s, Belbin found that effective teams were founded upon individual behaviours. The research was originally contrived to examine ways to control team dynamics; however, the researchers found that the difference between success and failure in a team was not based on intellect but on separate clusters of behaviour; each behaviour making a specific contribution to effective team working.

Belbin went on to identify nine team roles, each equally essential to the team and necessary to create a balance of roles. Of note, each identified role also displays some potential weaknesses which can interfere with team productivity, but which are tolerated because of the positives that role also brings to the team. (See the useful websites at the end of the chapter for more information on Belbin's work.)

Influence of social systems on teams

Teams do not work in isolation. In healthcare, they are often located in organisations or as subsets of other larger team structures, such as departments or divisions. These background factors need to be taken into consideration for a full analysis of team dynamics (personal relationships) and processes (actions directed toward a specific aim). The sociologist George Homans (1961) used a systemic model to describe what he determined as the *internal systems* facing *external systems*, and the impact of systems or feedback loops on team dynamics and, consequently, the effectiveness of teams.

An example of a system is the water cycle. Water vapour is condensed from the atmosphere into clouds. It falls onto the earth as rain or snow and is collected into some form of reservoir. Humans channel the water into homes, factories and buildings. It is then utilised and transformed into wastewater, which travels into rivers and seas to be evaporated back into the clouds, thus beginning the cycle all over again. At each stage, there are factors which influence the system, such as drought, over-usage and contamination. Equally, social systems can be affected by Political, Economic, Social, Technological, Legislative or Environmental factors and therefore indicate the complexity, interdependency and vulnerability of any system, as well as an ability to adapt to change. Understanding systems and how they work can have an impact on problem solving, team working and the management of change (see useful websites for more information on management application of systems thinking and PESTLE analyses).

While the importance of Homans' focus on individuals in small groups is now quoted less often, the fundamental findings of his work help to illuminate the factors that influence small-group functioning as a system, and the consequences of those interactions, such as the impact of the manager's leadership style and external organisational infrastructures. Homans considered the essential elements of a group system to be the activities, processes, interactions, interpersonal relationships and attitudes of team members toward the goals of the team. See Figure 3.1 for a contemporary version of Homans' conceptual scheme.

The conceptual feedback loop scheme Homans designed can help us to analyse groups and pinpoint problem areas when teams are ineffective. The importance of this work is to acknowledge that each action influences other parts of the process in a system, which is a major characteristic of general systems theory (famously illustrated by von Bertalanffy, 1968) and also of any small-group interaction. Homans' studies led to the development of social exchange theory and the premise that social interaction is based on the exchange of rewards.

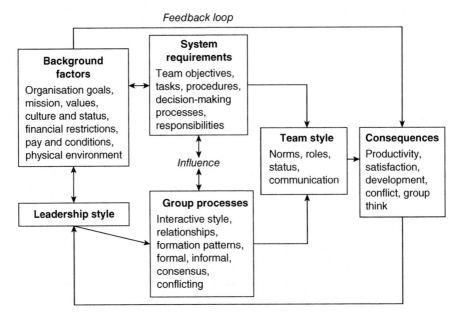

Figure 3.1 Homans' (1961) conceptual scheme of a small social system modified to reflect external and internal influences on consequences or effective outputs of a team in the twenty-first century.

Theory summary: Social exchange theory

This theory is based on establishing and sustaining reciprocity (equal exchange) in social relationships, or mutual gratification between individuals, and the comparison of alternatives. The theory relies on the assumption that humans are rational and willing to exchange items, either material or emotional, that are important to them for the benefit of other people. Integral concepts of the theory are the notions of justice and fairness. If the perceived costs of a relationship outweigh the benefits, the theory predicts that a person will leave the relationship. However, criticisms of the theory are that it favours an economic model, whereby all human interaction is likened to a process of cost–benefit analysis. Furthermore, there are opportunities for coercion and power tactics through the use of punishments and rewards if benefits are withdrawn. This is particularly evident in hierarchical or highly structured environments and groupings. The perceived effect of social obligations versus the amount of freedom of choice to exchange commodities can also negatively affect relationships. Understanding the intricacies of social exchange theory can help you understand social relationships in a team, when some people are more willing to help others, for example. (See the useful websites listed at the end of the chapter for further information.)

Creating effective team working

There is a lot of emphasis in the management literature on team-building activities to enhance team effectiveness by focusing on both task and relationship aspects of team working. The aims of team building are generally to:

- establish goals or specific objectives;
- clarify the values, purpose and functions of the team;
- allocate or re-allocate work roles and responsibilities;
- establish or revive communication patterns;
- clarify the group norms or expected behaviours of the team;
- complete a job of work;
- identify the decision-making processes, responsibilities and hierarchies to define inter-team relationships.

Team building starts at recruitment. Identifying the skills, both essential and desirable, which are needed when recruiting to a team, creates the opportunity for the manager, or leader, to complement and strengthen those skills already available to them and to fill skills gaps which will be of benefit to the team. This team building continues at short listing and interviewing, when the manager has the opportunity to first sift applicants for talent and then interview them to ensure their values are a good fit for the existing team (Foster, 2017).

Team-building strategies can be used to help integrate individuals into teams, for example through the training and introductions to the team undertaken at induction, making them function more effectively from the point at which they join the team. Team-building exercises may also require funding and time away from the work situation. Alternatively, the team leader can undertake an analysis of the team's functioning, if the team only needs fine tuning, through processes such as supervision and appraisal (see the useful websites at the end of the chapter for team-building ideas). Team leaders can also undertake an objective observation of team activities and then take this to team meetings for an open discussion. The team leader will need to take the emotional temperature of the team to decide if this will be appropriate (we discuss more about emotional intelligence, which will aid this process, in Chapter 5).

Activity 3.4   Reflection

Consider your own induction to a team or working environment and consider the value of the training offered as well as any opportunities to meet other staff. Consider whether the people undertaking the induction discussed the values, vision or goals of the organisation. If so, did this enable you to better understand the nature of the team you were joining.

Since this is based on your own thoughts and reflections, there is no specimen answer at the end of the chapter.

Where the leader has to intervene because a team is not functioning effectively, they will need to do some preparation aimed at analysing and defining the problems. This involves four steps:

1. Gathering information through different means, such as:

    (a) informal and formal discussions with individuals;

    (b) surveying the work done and comparing it to that which should be done;

    (c) reviewing notes from one-to-one sessions and personal development reviews/ appraisals;

    (d) team meetings;

    (e) team supervision.

2. Identifying the team's, and individuals within the teams', strengths and areas for development.

3. Creating a plan of action with the team.

4. Identifying time to work on the issues identified in steps 1 and 2 above, and in implementing the plan.

Background information can also be gathered about the structures of the organisation in which the team works. This includes the current work climate and culture (e.g. financial constraints), team goals and the professional setting (e.g. mental health, community nursing, interdisciplinary, stroke rehabilitation, infection control). It is important to consider the extent to which members work as autonomous individuals within the team, whether they are based in a unit or spread out over a geographical area, the complexity of roles and responsibilities, problem-solving styles, interpersonal relationships and relations with other groups in the organisation.

Sullivan and Decker (2009) suggest the following eight questions should be asked:

1. *To what extent does the team accept the goals of the organisation?*

2. *What, if any, hidden agendas interfere with the team's performance?*

3. *How effective is the team leadership?*

4. *To what extent do team members understand and accept their roles and responsibilities?*

5. *How does the team make a decision?*

6. *How does the team handle conflict? Are conflicts dealt with through avoidance or denial, force, accommodation, compromise, competition or collaboration?*

7. *What personal feelings do members have about each other?*

8. *To what extent do members trust and respect each other?*

All this takes time, and the leader will need to exercise diplomacy and tact when seeking answers to these questions. The leader also needs to be aware that the process of asking these questions may uncover some difficult truths about the team, or individuals within the team, which they will not be able to ignore.

Strategies for managing team problems

We have discussed how to create effective team working, and we go into more detail by studying different styles of leadership and management elsewhere in this text. It is, however, worth breaking here to consider the stages a manager might go through if they are experiencing issues within the nursing team.

Antai-Otong (1997) suggests the following stages:

If the member is not a team player:

- consider carefully whether or not you want the person on the team;
- interact with the member assertively;
- give the person an opportunity to provide feedback on problematic situations.

If communication with other team members is part of the problem:

- speak to the person one-to-one;
- listen actively when the person speaks, assessing verbal and non-verbal messages to identify any underlying issues or anxieties;
- avoid blaming and shaming, which tends to create defensiveness and arguments.

If the member seems to lack a sense of personal accountability:

- explain how failure to take responsibility affects the whole team (and give an example);
- without blaming or shaming, provide feedback from all team members.

If the team lacks clear goals:

- brainstorm activity to clarify short-term goals and develop an action plan with the team;
- strive for consensus regarding mission and goals;
- define member responsibilities;
- determine resources to accomplish goals (e.g. staffing expertise, financial, administrator support, time and equipment);
- periodically review team progress and achievements.

If team roles and boundaries are unclear:

- clarify role boundaries with the team's input;
- define all roles in the team, including the leader's;
- periodically review the team's staff or professional development needs.

Of course, experiencing problems with staff, and within teams, is not an issue confined to nursing teams and, as Ellis (2021b) points out, in these situations the first question any leader should ask is, 'am I the problem?'

Communication within the team

One of the most frequent causes of poor teamwork is inadequate or failing communication. A major problem in busy units, wards and departments is dealing with distractions if essential information is to be communicated. Most distractions are through sensory perceptions, such as poor lighting or background noise, talking, music, ringing phones and interruptions. Moving to a quieter environment, or agreeing a time to speak when all parties can concentrate, will help to minimise distractions. Team member anxieties around reporting, heavy workloads and keeping up to date can also be distracting.

Different levels of knowledge can create frustration between staff and misunderstandings over expectations if a standard of knowledge is not met. This requires a culture of openness in the team so that members feel free to ask questions and are not embarrassed to admit to not having specific information. It also requires the leader to act as the conductor, employing the different and varying skills of the team members in different ways, ensuring they understand their contribution and appreciate the contribution of others toward getting the job of work done.

Good communication in teams needs to be frequent and involve all staff members. When spontaneous decisions have to be made, individuals can feel left out of the loop. All organisational and planning decisions should be agreed by consensus. However, an understanding that, in exceptional circumstances, there may be no time to communicate, should also be agreed. Building in protected time or a mechanism to debrief the team on situations that fall outside the usual can help. We have seen examples of this during the coronavirus pandemic, where decisions which affected the work of healthcare teams had to be made and implemented with little or no notice, as well as the increasing recognition that the people involved in the provision of care require debriefing and support to help them come to terms with the challenges of the situation (Welch-Horan et al., 2021).

Differences in perception can misrepresent messages. The same message can be distorted through a lens of individual biases and preconceptions, sociocultural, ethnic and educational differences. Teams need to develop tolerance and awareness of how various team members see the world. This is best achieved through team meetings and encouraging team members to work in the same space where possible.

Distress, anxiety, heightened emotional states and certain personality traits, such as neuroticism, which is one of five key personality traits typified by excessive anxiety or indecision (Brewer, 2019), can interfere with message communications. As all members of any team are only human, home life stresses may be brought to the workplace. Team members need to feel safe to express their anxieties and have support from colleagues and the leader. However, if the stresses are interfering with effective working, occupational health support should be sought.

Dealing with meetings and committees

When you have a busy day ahead with many things on your to-do list, the last thing you may feel like spending time on is either going to a meeting or leading one. Meetings have a reputation for being boring and ineffective. But a well-led meeting can produce some very satisfying results and ensure everyone uses their time efficiently and purposively. Meetings are the processes by which organisations conduct their business through committee structures. There are different types of committees with distinct responsibilities and decision-making powers. Formal committees are part of the governance structures of an organisation and have different levels of authority and scope to make decisions. The highest level of committee structure within an organisation is board level (see useful websites for further information). The responsibilities and functions of any committee are outlined in their **terms of reference** along with the membership, frequency and **quorate** requirements (minimum required numbers attending for decisions to be made). Very often committees have subcommittees that are convened to deal with specific tasks or matters that need specialist and focused attention.

Other committees may have an advisory remit but no authority or power, although they may have a strong influence on decisions. Committees are also set up to undertake specific tasks to be completed in a defined time span. An example is to develop a proposal for service development. The committee may then be tasked with implementing the developments (often called a task and finish group) or, alternatively, charged with investigating problems that require recommendations to be sent to a formal committee for action. Another form of committee will monitor activities such as standards or quality enhancement (for example, an audit or service improvement committee).

At ward or unit level, the team meetings, where staff get together to discuss issues and problems and formulate local policies and procedures, are the focal point of work life. These meetings need to be seen as the pivotal place for decisions, discussions and forward planning to enhance the work environment and service delivery. It is the team leader's responsibility to ensure that the relevance and role of the meetings are understood and valued by team members. It should also be a time to enjoy being with colleagues who have a shared vision of their working lives. The value of human contact at meetings has never been better illustrated than during the coronavirus pandemic, when many meetings moved to the online environment.

Preparation, place and time, participation

Classically, the key to successful meetings has been to follow the three Ps: preparation, place and time and participation.

- *Preparation* is about clearly identifying the *purpose* of the meeting. Even if it is a short meeting, there should be an agenda with items to be discussed plainly stated and an indication as to whether the item is for discussion, decision or information.

The leader needs to think ahead about the agenda items and undertake pre-reading, so that they are ready to respond to questions and have potential solutions to problems ready, as well as an idea of delegated responsibilities if this is required.

- *Place and time*: advance information about venue and duration is vital. Meetings are work and not social gatherings, so an emphasis on getting things done and an action-oriented approach are needed to encourage effective use of time. Members will also think it worthwhile attending if their time is not wasted.

- *Participation*: your knowledge of team dynamics and the roles your team members play, whether nurturing or task-oriented, will be valuable in understanding how team members participate in the meeting. Their ability to contribute will also depend on their level of skills and knowledge. However, this could be detrimentally affected by the phenomenon known as **group think**, which is a particular concern if you have a philosophy of self-directedness in a group of experienced professionals. The ability to chair meetings, take notes if necessary, delegate activities and follow up on actions are key elements of an effective meeting.

The term 'Platform' might prove a useful addition to the list in the post pandemic working world, where many meetings have shifted online and people need not only to understand how to access the online platform, but also the required norms of behaviour attendant with being at a meeting, but not in a shared space.

Theory summary: From group think to team think

In the 1970s, social psychologist Irving Janis identified the phenomenon of group think, which happens when a group makes faulty decisions (Janis, 1972, 1982). This is due to pressures from within the group, whose members ignore alternatives and make irrational decisions that ignore the humanising factors present in other groups or sections of an organisation or community. When group members are from the same background, are insulated from outside influences, and there are no clear decision-making structures, they are particularly susceptible to group think. There are eight documented symptoms of group think:

1. An illusion of invulnerability creates excessive optimism that encourages taking extreme risks.
2. Belief in collective rationalisation – members discount warnings and do not reconsider their assumptions.
3. Belief in inherent morality – members believe in the rightness of their cause and therefore ignore the ethical or moral consequences of their decisions.
4. Stereotyped views of other groups lead to negative views of 'the enemy', which make effective responses to conflict seem unnecessary.
5. Direct pressure on dissenters involves putting members under pressure to avoid expressing arguments against any of the group's views.

6. Self-censorship means that doubts and deviations from the perceived group consensus are not expressed.
7. Illusion of unanimity – the majority view and judgements are assumed to be unanimous.
8. Self-appointed 'mind guards' involve members protecting the group and the leader from information that is problematic or contradictory to the group's cohesiveness, view and/or decisions.

When groups are tightly knit and under pressure to make decisions, irrational decisions are likely, as alternatives are not considered. Failure to discuss options and potential outcomes leads to carelessness and a need to achieve unanimity. The overall outcome is groups that have a low probability of successful decision-making.

To move toward 'team think', team leaders need to facilitate discussions in teams that are not reliant only on members of the team, by introducing observers to the team or other specialists to give a point of view. Dealing with dominant members, as discussed previously, and not putting the team under pressure, will also offset these effects. One of the main factors is always to consider alternative perspectives and the viewpoints or goals of other teams or activities in the organisation, to gain a wider viewpoint of how decisions fit into the whole picture before making final decisions.

Interdisciplinary team working

Up until now this chapter has focused on team working within a professional group or disciplinary area, although it is acknowledged that there are many different types of teams working within nursing. In health and social care today, there is an increasing need for professionals from different disciplines to work together to improve patient services. Nurses, physicians, dieticians, social workers, pharmacists, physiotherapists, administrators and technicians, among others, may all find themselves working together with a common aim but a different perspective on how to achieve this aim.

Activity 3.5   Evidence-based practice and research

Think about the different members of staff working in your most recent placement. Do you know what all of them do? If not, you might ask them next time you are in practice. Or you could ask your practice supervisor if you might spend some time with an individual from a different professional background. Consider the interactions you have witnessed between people from different professional disciplines and whether they might all share the same objectives as nurses. You might find it enlightening to attend an interdisciplinary, or multidisciplinary, team meeting as part of your development.

(Continued)

(Continued)

At the start of the chapter, you saw that outcome 5.4 requires the registered nurse to: *demonstrate an understanding of the roles, responsibilities and scope of practice of all members of the nursing and interdisciplinary team and how to make best use of the contributions of others involved in providing care.* You should analyse the contribution different members of the interdisciplinary team make in your placement area, note the role of each team member and discuss with your practice assessor how each person contributes to the holistic care of patients. You may want to make notes for your assessment portfolio.

There is no right or wrong answer to this activity.

Scaria (2016) notes how interprofessional working requires co-operation and a desire to work toward a common goal, yet there are many barriers that can prevent this from happening, including poor communication and diverse knowledge bases. They felt multidisciplinary working could develop by identifying areas of common ground, in particular around developing **care pathways**. To achieve effective interprofessional working, the role of the team leader is crucial in order to minimise professional rivalries and retain a central focus on patient need.

In common with all elements of good leadership, working with other professions requires that the leader is clear about the values of the team. In the care setting, this will mean a desire to achieve positive outcomes for patients or clients; what different professionals view as a positive outcome and how this is achieved is not as important as the fact that they all support achieving a positive outcome, as described by the patient.

The following is an account of a study to examine the effectiveness of a team and the multidisciplinary working processes.

Research summary: The impact of team processes on psychiatric case management

This is a study undertaken to identify the structures and interactions within community mental health teams that facilitate or impede effective teamwork and psychiatric case management. The view of the researchers was that effective case management requires close collaboration between case managers or care co-ordinators and other members of the multidisciplinary mental health team, yet there has been little research into this relationship. A multiple case study of seven UK community mental health teams was conducted between 1999 and 2001, using qualitative methods of participant observation, semi-structured interviews and document review. Factors were identified from the study that impacted on the ability of care co-ordinators to act effectively. These were *structure and procedures; disrespect and withdrawal; humour and undermining; safety and disclosure.*

Care co-ordination was enhanced when team structures and policies were in place and where team interactions were respectful. Where members felt disrespected or undermined, communication, information sharing and collaboration were impaired, with a negative impact on the care provided to service users. The researchers concluded that teams require clear operating procedures alongside trust and respect across the professions if there is to be open, safe and reflective participation.

Chapter summary

This chapter has given you an overview of how teams work, as well as how they do not work, and how you might improve your understanding of how the individuals who make up teams might work better together. There are strategies in the chapter to help you work more effectively with others in a leadership capacity or collegiate manner in teams. The chapter has only touched the surface and you are strongly recommended to access the useful websites or further reading to provide you with more detailed guidance.

Activities: Brief outline answers

Activity 3.2 Critical thinking (p52)

Teams utilise all of the skills of the people in the team and, because these skills complement each other and one person can pick up where another person's skills end, teams can solve more complex problems than individuals can manage alone. Because people have different skills, the breadth of work they can achieve in teams is increased, as is the complexity of the task which may be undertaken.

Activity 3.3 Reflection (p52)

Teams are not effective just because they are. Rather they are effective because the people within the teams want them to be, share common goals and values and put these into practice. When values are relegated to second place after targets, then the quality of the work of the team is affected, as described in the Francis report (2013).

Further reading

Grant, A and Goodman, B (2018) *Communication and Interpersonal Skills in Nursing* (4th edition). London: SAGE.

Two chapters deal with effective team working and the working environment – Chapter 5: Understanding Potential Barriers, and Chapter 7: The Environmental Context.

Jelphs, K, Dickinson, H and Miller, R (2016) *Working in Teams* (2nd edition). Bristol: Policy Press.

Chapter 1 is a useful introduction, while Chapter 2 has some things to say about interprofessional working.

Useful websites

www.acas.org.uk

Advisory, Conciliation and Arbitration Service (ACAS), has a number of resources relating to conflict in the workplace.

www.managementhelp.org/grp_skll/meetings/meetings.htm

Free Management Library information on preparing, planning, leading and evaluating meetings.

http://managementhelp.org/systems/systems.htm#anchor6759

Free Management Library on the development and application of systems theory to analyse problems and influence change management.

www.businessballs.com/teambuilding.htm

This site provides ideas for team building, organisational structures and also discussion around corporate social responsibility and ethical organisations.

www.belbin.com

Home page for Belbin's team role theory, role descriptors and explanations of the theory.

www.infed.org/thinkers/george_homans.htm

Provides background to the work of the sociologist George Homans and the development of social exchange theory.

www.the-happy-manager.com/tips/pestle-analysis

A short and clear overview of the PESTLE analysis tool.

Chapter 4 Working with individuals in teams

This chapter will address the following platforms and proficiencies:

Platform 1: Being an accountable professional

Registered nurses act in the best interests of people, putting them first and providing nursing care that is person-centred, safe and compassionate. They act professionally at all times and use their knowledge and experience to make evidence-based decisions about care. They communicate effectively, are role models for others, and are accountable for their actions. Registered nurses continually reflect on their practice and keep abreast of new and emerging developments in nursing, health and care.

At the point of registration, the registered nurse will be able to:

1.5　understand the demands of professional practice and demonstrate how to recognise signs of vulnerability in themselves or their colleagues and the action required to minimise risks to health.

1.10　demonstrate resilience and emotional intelligence and be capable of explaining the rationale that influences their judgments and decisions in routine, complex and challenging situations.

Platform 4: Providing and evaluating care

Registered nurses take the lead in providing evidence-based, compassionate and safe nursing interventions. They ensure that care they provide and delegate is person-centred and of a consistently high standard. They support people of all ages in a range of care settings. They work in partnership with people, families and carers to evaluate whether care is effective and the goals of care have been met in line with their wishes, preferences and desired outcomes.

(Continued)

(Continued)

At the point of registration, the registered nurse will be able to:

4.14 demonstrate and apply an understanding of what is important to people and how to use this knowledge to ensure their needs for safety, dignity, privacy, comfort and sleep can be met, acting as a role model for others in providing evidence-based person-centred care.

Platform 5: Leading and managing nursing care and working in teams

Registered nurses provide leadership by acting as a role model for best practice in the delivery of nursing care. They are responsible for managing nursing care and are accountable for the appropriate delegation and supervision of care provided by others in the team including lay carers. They play an active and equal role in the interdisciplinary team, collaborating and communicating effectively with a range of colleagues.

At the point of registration, the registered nurse will be able to:

5.4   demonstrate an understanding of the roles, responsibilities and scope of practice of all members of the nursing and interdisciplinary team and how to make best use of the contributions of others involved in providing care.

5.6   exhibit leadership potential by demonstrating an ability to guide, support and motivate individuals and interact confidently with other members of the care team.

5.7   demonstrate the ability to monitor and evaluate the quality of care delivered by others in the team and lay carers.

5.9   demonstrate the ability to challenge and provide constructive feedback about care delivered by others in the team, and support them to identify and agree individual learning needs.

Platform 6: Improving safety and quality of care

Registered nurses make a key contribution to the continuous monitoring and quality improvement of care and treatment in order to enhance health outcomes and people's experience of nursing and related care. They assess risks to safety or experience and take appropriate action to manage those, putting the best interests, needs and preferences of people first.

At the point of registration, the registered nurse will be able to:

6.8   demonstrate an understanding of how to identify, report and critically reflect on near misses, critical incidents, major incidents and serious adverse events in order to learn from them and influence their future practice.

Chapter aims

After reading this chapter, you will be able to:

- understand the significance of the concepts 'responsibility' and 'accountability' in relation to individuals in teams;
- evaluate the factors affecting the delegation of work within a team;
- evaluate the role of personal development plans (PDPs) for an individual in a team;
- understand the relevance of individual, organisational, generational and cultural differences to team working.

Introduction

In this chapter, topics such as individual roles, responsibility and accountability, with reference to the NMC *Code* (NMC, 2018b) will be discussed, along with techniques for successful delegation. PDPs, performance appraisal and staff development principles will be explored. Cultural and generational differences will be discussed. Employment issues such as health and safety legislation and risk management will be included in this chapter. Recruitment, selection and retention of staff will be covered briefly in Chapter 7. In addition, you will find it helpful to look at the NMC (2018b) *Code*, which has specific guidance for nurses, midwives and nursing associates working with others. Some key areas covered in this guidance include:

1. Communicate clearly.

2. Work co-operatively.

3. Share your skills, knowledge and experience for the benefit of people receiving care and your colleagues.

4. Be accountable for your decisions to delegate tasks and duties to other people.

Activity 4.1   Evidence-based practice and research

Go to the NMC web page (**www.nmc-uk.org**) and review the underpinning principles of these themes proposed by the NMC.

These principles and themes are further discussed throughout this chapter.

The NMC (2018a) *Future Nurse: Standards of Proficiency for Registered Nurses* and *The Code* (2018b) place considerable emphasis on team working and the responsibility of both the individual within the team and the team leader. In this chapter we will be focusing on the leadership role in supporting, developing and challenging individuals in the team.

Individual roles, responsibility and accountability

In the previous chapter we looked at the many different forms and types of team, and the ways in which teams can work together. In this chapter we will be concentrating on the individuals in the team and will begin by looking at roles and responsibilities. Each team will have a defined purpose, indicated in the two scenarios below.

Scenarios: Different examples of teams

Team A is brought together for a short-term activity such as the length of a shift. This could be a band 5 nurse caring for six patients in a section of a ward, possibly, and depending on the acuity of the needs of the patients or the seriousness of the illnesses, with another band 5 colleague and two healthcare assistants (HCAs) from 7 a.m. to 3 p.m.

Team B is a multidisciplinary team convened to work together for a longer duration to implement a new service initiative to improve patient care. In this example it is a project group to ensure patients receive dignified care.

Within each of these teams an individual team member will have a role or a part to play in completing a task and in the overall remit of the team and will be responsible for various actions. It is worth reminding ourselves of the meaning of the word 'responsible' and how that relates to the concept of accountability.

Activity 4.2   Critical thinking

Write out your definitions of 'responsible' and 'accountable' without referring to a dictionary. Think about the differences between the two concepts.

Then think about what the difference is for those who are leading teams and for those who are being led.

Further guidance is given on this activity at the end of the chapter.

The next step is to ensure team members understand their responsibilities in relation to a task. A team leader is expected to assign responsibility for activities, and this can become a minefield of emotions and hurt feelings if communicated inappropriately or to a person with the wrong skill set or knowledge. We will discuss this in more detail later in the chapter when we discuss delegation, but in this discussion we are focusing on conveying a sense of responsibility to complete team work successfully. Conveying a sense of responsibility requires clear thinking and communication about what is expected, as well as checking progress throughout the task. If this is not done, leaders, by failing to lead, are the ones responsible for less than satisfactory results and cannot hold team members accountable for any shortfalls. To ensure responsibilities are understood and carried out:

- identify the appropriate team member with the skills and knowledge to carry out the task;
- ensure resources are available for the task to be completed or advise, and empower, the team member on how to obtain resources;
- explain and assign the task;
- identify the level of support to be given to the team member (e.g. is the person novice or experienced?);
- set the standards;
- check progress;
- make sure the standards are met and the task completed.

At team level the same rules apply. The team needs to be put together so that the skills and abilities needed to undertake the task are all collected in one place. Team members need an understanding of the task and their role in undertaking the task, as well as the resources to do it. They will also need support and progress checks from their manager.

Delegation

As a team leader you can only delegate those tasks for which you are responsible. As we have seen above, the delegator remains accountable for the task, whereas the delegate is accountable to the delegator and has responsibilities for the task being assigned.

Delegation is a means of dividing up the workload in a team. It is also a way for leaders to help team members develop or enhance their abilities and skills. It can promote team working, foster collaboration and increase the amount of work achievable in a given time when compared with a person working alone. Delegation is also a good tool for preparing people for the next step in their career; in this sense it can prove to be very motivational. As research has demonstrated, however, it is not a skill all nurses have on qualification. It requires work to become good at it (Magnusson et al., 2017).

Delegation is not a means of escaping tasks or responsibilities that leaders do not want. Nor is it work or task allocation. Allocating tasks is to transfer a task from one person to another, whereas delegation gives someone the authority to carry out a task in place of the person who would normally undertake that task. By transferring authority, the person has the right to act and is empowered to undertake the task (i.e. this could be to ask others to undertake subtasks as part of the overall activity). This difference should be made explicit to the delegatee when a task is delegated.

Scenarios

Let's return to the scenario of Team B. Within this group there are representatives from different wards in a hospital, as the initiative is to be undertaken across the organisation. The team also includes representatives of different disciplines. Once a plan of action has been agreed, to ensure dignity is implemented on the wards, the representatives will go back to their bases and initiate changes in the ward to bring about a successful outcome. They will need the collaboration of their peers, subordinates and, possibly, seniors to carry out subtasks. They may be experts in change-management strategies and be able to charm the birds from the trees, but they will also need the authority to undertake this task and have that recognised by the teams they are going to be working with. Multidisciplinary workers may have to work with professions other than their own. To be successful, they will also need their personal skills and the support of the authority invested in the group to bring about these changes. The authority invested in the project group, probably by a senior member of the directorate or division, will provide the legitimate authority for the project to carry out adjustments in the wards.

In the case of Team A, where tasks are being divided among the team, the aim is to assign relevant activities to the appropriately qualified, or grade, of staff. The team leader will have the authority to assign the tasks and the responsibility to match activities to grade or competence. However, the team member has the responsibility for his or her own activities and the care of the patient.

Delegation decisions

Who to delegate to and how to delegate are, for the novice, quite daunting decisions. There are several potential competing thoughts and feelings impacting these decisions, such as:

- guilt in asking someone else to do a job that you are qualified or competent to undertake;
- reluctance to delegate if you think you can do a task better or more quickly;
- having to ask someone you are equal to in grade or who you haven't worked with before.

Activity 4.3 Reflection

Consider the last time someone delegated responsibility to you. How did you feel? What reasons might you have had for wanting, or not wanting, to do the task? Did you feel you had the authority to see the task through? Did the person delegating the task make you feel they still had some accountability for how the task turned out?

Further guidance is given on this activity at the end of the chapter.

Working with skill mix

Changing care needs and priorities mean care leaders have to get used to thinking about and adapting to the changing **skill mix** in their teams. In NHS acute care settings, increasing numbers of HCAs will be working alongside qualified nurses undertaking whole-patient care and not just tasks such as personal care and observations of temperature, pulse and respirations (Cornish and Holloway, 2019). Most hospital HCAs are employed at band 3, and you may want to request a copy of the generic job description for this grade to understand its scope of practice. The job description should link to the NHS Agenda for Change band (NHS Employers, n.d.a) and the NHS Knowledge and Skills Framework national clinical grading criteria (NHS Employers, n.d.b). Increasingly, HCAs are taking up nursing associate roles, as many have completed a specialised foundation degree in healthcare. Nursing associates are usually employed at Agenda for Change band 4, a step up from the grading of an HCA, but below that of a registered nurse. It would be worth your while looking at the difference between these various grades as well as the difference in the roles and responsibilities of a nursing associate and a registered nurse.

In addition, some HCAs will have achieved National Vocational Qualifications (NVQs) at level 3 or 4, now more often called the Qualifications and Credit Framework (QCF). NVQs and QCFs are competency-based qualifications and there are five levels within a structure called the Regulated Qualifications Framework (RQF). The RQF is an index of qualifications by level and number of credits, and makes it simple to compare similar qualifications which are awarded under different names. See the useful websites at the end of the chapter for more information.

In mixed teams providing acute care to adult patients, qualified nurses will need to delegate care to nursing associates and HCAs and other non-professionally registered staff, such as domestic or ancillary personnel. In community settings, health visitors delegate care to nursery nurses and band 5 nurses (staff nurses) who undertake some developmental screening. In some teams, such as intermediate care in the community, community practitioners are band 5 staff nurses working with specialist community practice home nurses. In acute mental health settings, assistant practitioners work with registered mental health nurses. In childcare, nursery nurses work with staff nurses, and in learning disability settings, registered learning disability nurses work with nursing assistants.

All this points to the fact that the leader must be aware not only of the work which needs to be done by the team, but also the skill sets available from within the team. Knowing the team and the skill mix within the team will enable the leader to make appropriate decisions about task delegation and will help to promote effective care provision.

Activity 4.4   Evidence-based practice and research

Go online and find the NHS Knowledge and Skills Framework. Take the opportunity to review not only the six core dimensions of the framework, but also some of the summary, or generic, post outlines. Doing this will enable you to understand what is required of different staff roles and give you some insight into what is appropriate to delegate and what is not.

Since the answers to this activity depend on what you search, there is no specimen answer at the end of the chapter.

Enabling staff development through delegation

By delegating tasks and responsibilities to other members of the team, opportunities can be provided for staff development, increased job satisfaction and promotion. It has been understood for some considerable time that one of the key motivators of people in the workplace lies in giving them responsibility to undertake tasks which stretch them professionally (Herzberg, 1959). People also have a need to undertake tasks which they see as worthwhile and which might contribute to their advancement, both personally and professionally (Herzberg, 1959). It should be clear by now that one of the criteria for role satisfaction for all team members must be that they are doing something that aligns with their values. Factors such as a positive organisational culture encourage delegation, as well as the expression of personal qualities that engender co-operation and a willingness to collaborate, the appropriate use of resources (equipment and learning environment) and appropriate supervision or guidance for the task.

Selecting the right person to delegate to requires a corresponding leadership style. It is often assumed that delegation is a management role; however, recognising the talents and strengths of individuals and working to meet their developmental stages require leadership qualities. Kotter (1990) recognised this and developed a scheme for matching the appropriate leadership style to the individual's levels of commitment and competence. This enables leaders to draw out the best in their team members and identify where development needs to take place. Table 4.1 outlines an adaptation of Kotter's ideas. We discuss coaching in Chapter 6.

The rules for delegation are the same no matter what the task or the grade of the person being delegated to:

1. *Identify the task to be delegated.*

2. *Identify the person(s) to be delegated to.*

3. *Ensure that the person(s) being delegated to have the ability to undertake the task.*

4. *Ensure the reasons for the delegation are understood.*

5. *Ensure the expected outcome and time frame are understood.*

6. *Ensure resources and authority to see through task are in place.*

7. *Ensure the recipient(s) of the delegated task are supported.*

8. *Give feedback on the results of the delegation.*

(Ellis, 2015, p71)

Developmental level of individuals	Appropriate leadership style
Low competence – high commitment	Directing
Some competence – low commitment	Coaching
High competence – variable commitment	Supporting
High competence – high commitment	Delegating

Table 4.1   Matching individual levels of competence and motivation for tasks with leadership style

Source: Adapted from Kotter (1990).

Personal development plans

We have just talked about developing staff, so it would seem timely to introduce the topic of development planning. The PDP (sometimes called individual development plan or staff review) is intended to help employees enhance their existing skills or knowledge and develop new skills to fulfil an existing role. If responsibilities have increased, the PDP may be a tool used to indicate that an individual should be promoted to a higher grade. Alternatively, it can be used to identify a role at a grade equivalent to a previous role. In NHS settings, the PDP should be carried out annually and is a method of ensuring staff maintain their skills and knowledge to perform their roles.

The PDP provides a framework for:

- prioritising developmental support;
- planning related activities, such as attending study days, seminars or courses, in an appropriate sequence and within agreed timescales;
- monitoring progress within those timescales;

- evaluating outcomes in terms of skills, knowledge and expertise;
- developing individual career plans and identifying organisational succession plans.

As a student you may have completed a PDP that looks at your personal growth and development during your course. As a newly qualified nurse you will be expected to follow a period of preceptorship, which will give you the opportunity to identify areas you want to concentrate on during your preceptorship to extend your confidence in specific skills and knowledge. As you progress in experience and seniority, you may be involved in undertaking PDPs for other staff, and you would be advised to look out for any training being offered, as all organisations have a slightly different emphasis on how they conduct the PDP process. As a registered practitioner you will be required to maintain your professional knowledge to remain on the NMC register. In order to meet the criteria for revalidation, as a registered nurse you will have to demonstrate that you have undertaken (NMC, 2017):

- 450 practice hours, or 900 if renewing as both a nurse and midwife;
- 35 hours of CPD including 20 hours of participatory learning;
- five pieces of practice-related feedback;
- five written reflective accounts;
- reflective discussion;
- health and character declaration;
- professional indemnity arrangement;
- confirmation.

The practice element can be met through administrative, supervisory, teaching, research and managerial roles, as well as providing direct patient care.

Activity 4.5   Reflection

Look at the learning objectives you set with your practice assessor at the start of your last placement. Consider how the allocation of work which you undertook allowed you to meet the targets for development which you set. If you are newly qualified, you might like to do this activity with your preceptor or line manager, considering how your skills sets are growing to help meet the needs of the service in which you are working. These reflections are good practice for reflective discussions and accounts you will need to undertake for revalidation.

As this answer is based on your own observation, there is no outline answer at the end of the chapter.

Performance appraisal

Redshaw (2008) investigated the role and extent of appraisal in nursing. At the time, only six out of ten staff in the NHS received a formal appraisal. While more recent data on staff appraisal rates in the NHS are hard to come by, it is apparent that about 85 per cent of staff working in the NHS would agree that they always know what their 'work responsibilities are' (NHS Survey Coordination Centre, 2021). There is a distinction between appraisal – the judgement and assessment of the worth or value of an employee's performance at work – and personal development – a process of mutually planning (between staff member and senior staff in the organisation) supporting activities for individuals to undertake their role in the workplace. Appraisal does not always have a good press, as staff can feel that it is a waste of time or does not measure accurately their contribution to the work. Alternatively, some staff want to know how they are performing and to have some measure of performance as a yardstick to improve, for their own satisfaction or to progress in their career or work roles. Chapter 7 gives more information about performance appraisal.

There are different forms of appraisal scheme: top-down (the most common), self-appraisal and peer appraisal, upward appraisal where the appraiser reports on management's performance (the least common) and multi-rater appraisal, which is usually in the form of 360-degree feedback about an individual from a variety of peers, subordinates, external and internal appraisers and superiors – that is, everyone within the sphere of influence of an individual staff member.

The objective of appraisal is to identify and reward performance. If this is not achieved in practice, the scheme will lack merit. If there is an appraisal system alongside a personal development-planning scheme, the allocation of rewards can undermine the personal developmental aspects, as the emphasis will be on organisational aims and outputs. There are also concerns about the subjectivity of making appraisals that can be influenced by personal attributes of the appraiser or employee and environmental or situational factors, such as individual health, organisational changes and the time it takes to complete appraisals.

Support for staff – including performance review – can raise standards in the workplace. However, the quest for better performance has not always been accompanied by a better system of appraisal. According to Redshaw (2008), the most important process for improved performance is not to set goals and order staff to achieve them, but to improve relationships so that staff feel highly valued and have a sense of belonging. This idea reflects one of the ideas expressed in Chapter 2, when we identified that one of the key functions of the transformational leader is to set the vision for the team, an action which is known to motivate and inspire team members.

Conflicts, lack of understanding of the aims of the process, and mutual distrust will have a negative effect on the appraisal process, resulting in staff finding it difficult to accept criticism and feedback. This, in turn, will have a negative impact on staff performance. This is especially relevant in team-based work, where the style of the leader can influence colleagues' performance and attitudes toward appraisal. Another factor is the way in which feedback is handed to employees. Giving feedback can be challenging, and managers need good communication skills to ensure feedback is constructive and helpful. Feedback that is focused on blame damages self-confidence, whereas construc-tive criticism to recognise and improve poor performance is appropriate.

One way to think about the distinction between performance and appraisal, and the call from Redshaw to improve relationships, is to take the view that as appraisal only happens once a year, it may be too late, or too slow, in addressing issues in the work-place. A good relationship with staff is an ongoing thing and will reap rewards for the manager, and the staff member, throughout the whole of the year.

Case study: Ensuring adequate nutrition

The setting is a busy acute female medical ward. In a six-bedded bay, Mary, a slight 72-year-old who was originally admitted with unstable type 2 diabetes, is waiting to be discharged home. Although the ward staff have told her she won't be leaving until after lunch, Mary has had her bags packed since 7 a.m. as she is keen to leave the ward. Mary is a quiet and undemanding person who rarely complains. The band 5 team leader for the shift, Sandy, passes by the bed and sees that Mary has been provided with her lunch of soup and a sandwich. Nutrition is an important part of Mary's recovery plan to treat her diabetes, and also to help her restore her body mass index to within normal limits. Mary should be having fortified soups and not the usual soup, as she has been given in this instance, from the hospital menu. Fortified soups are available for patients in the ward kitchen. Sandy has spoken to the HCAs and ward hostess before about ensur-ing that Mary has fortified soups and that she receives reinforcing messages, when she has her meals, of the relevance and importance of maintaining her nutrition once she is at home. Sandy believes the HCAs are capable of giving health education as well as ensuring patients receive the appropriate nutrition. This would be in line with the NHS Knowledge and Skills Framework section on health and well-being and appropriate for an HCA to undertake. She also believes that the HCA, Joanna in this case, should have responsibility for ensuring the ward hostess provides the correct soup and that Joanna should monitor this. Sandy resolves to speak to the HCA to provide feedback on her performance and what she expects the HCA's role to be in this respect.

Evaluation and feedback are not the same thing (Jug et al., 2018). If we regard feedback as an ongoing process which is linked to staff development and evalua-tion as a final sign off, as a student might have at the end of a placement, it is obvious that they need to be approached differently. For the most part, exchanges between managers and staff should be feedback based, as they form part of an ongoing dialogue. Leaving criticism until an annual appraisal risks not allowing the staff member the time to address any deficits and potentially could cause harm to a patient as a result. Hardavella et al. (2017) suggest the following principles when giving feedback:

1. *Plan what you will say*

2. *Be contemporaneous, do it immediately after an event*

3. *Consider what it is you are trying to achieve*

4. *Usually one-to-one is best*

5. *Start with the simplest issues*

6. *Be specific about what you are referring to*

7. *Encourage the person to reflect*

8. *Watch the body language*

9. *Reflect after the feedback about what went well and what might have gone better*

Activity 4.6   Decision-making

Imagine that you are Sandy, the band 5 staff nurse on this shift, who is leading the team. Using the principles suggested by Hardavella et al. (2017), how would you go about providing feedback to Joanna? When would you give her the feedback?

Further guidance is given on this activity at the end of the chapter.

Individual, cultural and generational differences

Working with individuals in teams, the team leader will encounter individual differences in the team members that have to be acknowledged and worked with to ensure effective working relationships. In Chapter 1, we examined different roles that individuals assume in a team by individual differences. The chapter concentrates on the individual traits and personality that a person has. In Chapter 3, we had a brief look at these characteristics and now we can further explore personal characteristics that fall within the 'big five personality theory'.

Research summary: Five-factor model of personality

In 1991, Barrick and Mount reported on a study that they undertook to examine the relationships between workplace roles and individual personality characteristics, defined in the 'big five personality theory' or 'five-factor model of personality', as it is known theoretically. The personality dimensions are:

(Continued)

(Continued)

1. extroversion;
2. emotional stability;
3. agreeableness;
4. conscientiousness;
5. openness to experience.

These were matched to three job performance criteria (job proficiency, training proficiency and personnel data – i.e. age, time in occupation) for five occupational groups (professionals such as teachers, nurses and doctors; police; managers; sales; skilled/semi-skilled occupations).

The results of their analysis indicated that one dimension of personality, conscientiousness, showed consistent relations with all job performance criteria for all occupational groups. For the remaining personality dimensions, the correlations varied by occupational group and professional criteria.

Extroversion was a valid predictor for two occupations involving social interaction: managers and sales (across criterion types). Also, both openness to experience and extroversion were valid predictors of the training proficiency criterion (i.e. those persons who had a role as educators, and this was across all professions in the study). Other personality dimensions were also found to be valid predictors for some occupations and some criterion types, but the correlation between the occupation and criterion was small.

Overall, the results illustrated the benefits of using the five-factor model of personality to predict suitability for job performance. The findings were thought to have numerous implications for research and practice, especially in the subfields of personnel selection, training and development and performance appraisal. This means that there is some substance to the theory that certain personal characteristics are better suited to certain occupational roles.

Organisational culture

Another factor to influence individual behaviour in teams is cultural mores. Culture is not so much about what an organisation does; rather, in the sense we are thinking about it in this book, culture is about how staff experience their place of work (Handy, 2020). The philosophies, social and historical background to an organisation all shape the prevailing culture. In addition, practices within an organisation that are derived from leadership or management style have an enormous impact (Garcia et al., 2017). Examples include whether an organisation is people- or task-oriented; if there is an emphasis on control and command; the extent of tolerance to risk taking; if there is a reward culture or a blame culture; the manner in which an organisation responds to change – rapidly or at snail's pace – and finally, the extent to which an individual willingly signs up to the philosophy of the organisation.

Activity 4.7   Reflection

Think about the most recent teams you have been associated with. From the descriptions above, how would you describe them? Why do you think they were as they were? Did the culture of the team change when they faced a challenge? Why was that?

As this answer is based on your own observation, there is no outline answer at the end of the chapter.

Cultural diversity

The other aspect of culture is the sociological phenomenon of culture, which affects our lives in a complex and multifaceted manner in our culturally diverse society. To work collaboratively in teams, nurses have to understand and respect unfamiliar behaviour patterns and attitudes without dismissing or devaluing them. Yet, this diversity needs to be harnessed to be effective and to meet patients' needs. Grant and Goodman (2018) consider the relevance of focusing on cultural diversity and communication, as this is often the first barrier to overcome.

There are thought to be four cultural dimensions along which cultures differ in the workplace:

1. directness – getting to the point ↔ implying the messages;
2. hierarchy – following orders ↔ engaging in debate;
3. consensus – dissenting is accepted ↔ unanimity is needed;
4. individualism – individual winners are acceptable ↔ team effectiveness is paramount.

Different attitudes to authority, culturally embedded notions of authority and power, perceptions of gender stereotypes and acceptance of directness or expectations of hidden meanings in communications all influence these cultural dimensions. A team leader will need to be observant to recognise at which point of these dimensions individuals are expected to behave in the team and how each individual will be interpreting these dimensions, depending on their social and cultural background and the norms they are accustomed to. In addition, the philosophy of the organisation and the nature of the tasks undertaken (e.g. the perceived status of those tasks) will have an influence.

Generational differences

Every generation is affected by the time in which it grows up. Influences such as economic (e.g. post Second World War thriftiness), political (e.g. Thatcherism and individualistic political policies), social events (e.g. Bob Geldof's Live Aid concerts), feminist ideology and technological advances will play a significant part in forming the context for attitudes to be formed about work. While the cusp years can vary depending on the individual, here's how the generations are typically described:

- traditionalists or veterans: born before 1946;
- baby boomers: born between 1946 and 1964;
- generation X: born between 1965 and 1980;
- generation Y or millennials: born between 1980 and 1996;
- generation Z: born after 1996;

Patterson (2005) has gathered together observations from her work as an organisational psychologist and the business management literature to assemble impressions of the main characteristics associated with generations since the early part of the last century (Table 4.2) with adaptions to include generation Z (Chicca and Shellenbarger, 2018).

Traditionalists (1925–1945)	Baby boomers (1946–1964)	Generation X (1965–1980)	Millennials (1981 to 2000)	Generation Z
Practical	Optimistic	Sceptical	Hopeful	Independent
Patient, loyal and hardworking	Teamwork and co-operation	Self-reliant	Meaningful work	Confident
Respectful of authority	Ambitious	Risk taking	Diversity and change valued	Ambitious
Rule followers	Workaholic	Balances work and personal life	Technology-savvy	Digital native

Table 4.2 Defining work characteristics

Source: Adapted from Patterson (2005) and Chicca and Shellenbarger (2018).

While not everyone will fall into a defined category, taking note of generational diversity is important, as intergenerational lack of understanding of generational mores might impede working progress, teamwork and ideas for service improvement. For example, a baby boomer manager may not be familiar with social networking and the impact technologies have had on social relationships. The manager's ideas on how relationships are communicated and sustained might involve paper notices on notice boards, whereas the millennial team members will be likely to expect messages to be posted on a social networking site or perhaps communicated via a text messaging platform.

Research summary: Generational differences

Smola and Sutton (2002) surveyed 350 baby boomers and generation Xers in 1974 and 1999 and found an overall change in work values as generations matured, such as giving work a lower priority in life and placing less value on feeling a sense of pride at work. In particular, the younger women tend to question workplace expectations more often, such as long work hours or taking work home, and they are often more open about their parenting obligations and commitments. The study also found generational differences. For example, generation Xers report less loyalty to their companies, wanting to be promoted more quickly and being more 'me-oriented' than baby boomers. It is suggested that such differences are, in part, accounted for by workers' values shifting as they age. However, other researchers suggest that generational differences may not be a good indicator of how people feel, with actual age perhaps being a better indicator of this (Parry and Urwin, 2017).

Working in teams can cause clashes between individuals in the workplace. Baby boomers, traditionalists, generation Xers and millennials all represent different cultural norms as far as respecting tradition, social manners, speaking frankly about personal issues and attitudes to hierarchy are concerned. The generations will respond to change in different ways – fear of change can be expressed in one way if it results from being too used to certain ways of doing things, and in another way completely if it results from immaturity and insecurity. Baby boomers may find traditionalists inflexible, and may themselves be perceived as self-absorbed in return. Generation Xers, on the other hand, may find themselves criticised for being cynical and negative while seeing baby boomers as having their own conventional rigidity, and millennials as spoiled upstarts. Such clashes may be reduced if there are opportunities for facilitated discussion in team meetings, helping the various participants to explore the benefits and disadvantages of different approaches to working methods. A team leader will have the role of encouraging effective listening within the team, reducing ambiguity and misunderstandings, supporting the sharing of expertise and recognition of individuals' contributions to the team. It is helpful if the various generational groups can be encouraged to understand why each might respond in a particular fashion, and how patients might benefit in each case.

This approach is even more useful in interdisciplinary teams if misunderstandings are to be avoided. Team members can then work toward seeking a balance between building on traditional procedures and supporting newer ideas to blend the different work ethics of the generational groups.

According to Patterson (2005), effective, or similar, messages are for:

- traditionalists: 'Your experience is respected' or 'It is valuable to hear what has worked in the past';
- baby boomers: 'You are valuable, worthy' or 'Your contribution is unique and important to our success';

- generation Xers: 'Let's explore some options outside of the box' or 'Your technical expertise is a big asset';
- millennials: 'You will have an opportunity to collaborate with other bright, creative people' or 'You have really rescued this situation with your commitment'.

What this research shows, and indeed what comes out from the research of Parry and Urwin (2017), is that the important message for the leader is that different people view the world in different ways. This will mean that differing members of a team will have different needs and wants, as well as different abilities, and being aware of, and responding to, this in an appropriate way will mean the manager will get the most from individual team members and from the team as a whole.

This might remind you of the Johari window (Luft and Ingham, 1955) in Chapter 1, which presents to us some thoughts about the correlation between how we see ourselves and how other people see us. We said on p14 that 'there is great potential for us as individuals to lack understanding of ourselves as much as there is potential for other people not to understand us'. The message for the manager is that a good part of their role is learning to understand people and learning to use that understanding to get the best from them.

Chapter summary

This chapter has given you an overview of how teams work, what influences the behaviours of individuals within teams, and how you might better understand the way in which individuals in teams work together. There are strategies to help you work more effectively with others in a leadership capacity or collegiate manner in teams. The chapter has only touched the surface and you are strongly recommended to access the useful websites or further reading for more detailed guidance.

Activities: Brief outline answers

Activity 4.2 Critical thinking (p72)

The term 'responsible' can be understood from two perspectives:

1. being the cause of something, usually something wrong or disapproved of;
2. being answerable to someone for an action or the successful carrying out of a duty.

In a team, the team member has responsibility for carrying out an activity to the standard required by the team leader. To avoid perspective number 1 above, where misunderstandings, inaccuracies and disappointments may have occurred, the required standard should be explained to the person who is responsible for the task. In this situation it is the team leader's responsibility to be clear about what is expected in a task and the team member's responsibility to accomplish the task. Spending time explaining to a team member what is required can save time later and enables the team member to carry out the task up to the level required. It may be a peer who is in the team and, in this case, it would be helpful to clarify that both of you are working toward the same goal or outcome. If it is a subordinate or someone with untested skills or knowledge of the situation, an example or demonstration may be necessary to indicate the standard required for the task.

The term 'accountable' can be understood from two perspectives:

1. The obligations to report, explain or justify a behaviour or activity that has taken place and take responsibility for this activity. In this sense, a person is answerable to, or responsible to, another person, organisation or professional body for the way an activity has been undertaken. A key factor here is the word obligation, which can be interpreted as the legal responsibility or employment responsibility of the grade in which a person is employed. In this sense, it is accepting ownership for the results, or lack thereof. For example, a nurse is accountable to their employer, through their contract, and the NMC by virtue of their registration.

2. The capability of explaining why something has taken place (i.e. to give an account of something with reasons and/or evidence). In nursing, we more often use the first perspective rather than the second perspective, as the concept of accountability is blended with responsibility. Therefore, the team leader is accountable to the employer, with the responsibility for carrying out the task through the activities of the team members. The team members are accountable to the team leader and have responsibility to the team leader to carry out the required activity. However, the second perspective may be drawn upon if a person is required to give an account of the failure or success of a task.

Activity 4.3 Reflection (p75)

You may have wanted to do the task because it made you feel special, it may have been a good learning opportunity, or because you just wanted to be helpful. Reasons you might not have wanted to undertake the task include a lack of confidence, fear of failure or a dislike of taking responsibility. As a student you may have felt that you did not have the skills to do what is asked, but you should be learning them. Again, as a student delegated a task, the registered nurse should make it plain that they are accountable for the outcome, while you remain responsible for what you are doing.

Activity 4.6 Decision-making (p81)

The points you make may include the following:

1. Importance and rationale for nutrition in:

   (a) treatment of type 2 diabetes

   (b) weight maintenance.

2. Importance of health education information about maintaining diet when patient goes home.

3. Ensure the ward hostess gives the correct type of soup to Mary, by monitoring delivery.

4. Ensure Mary drinks the soup, even though she is keen to go home and not make a fuss.

5. Has Joanna had any additional training in diet and nutrition, and in particular with type 2 diabetes? If not, is there a training day coming up soon that she could attend?

6. Is Joanna comfortable monitoring the ward hostess? Does she see this as part of her role and her work in the team on this section of the ward? If not, explain that you have this expectation and you will support Joanna to do this by mentioning this as the expectation for all HCAs in the next team meeting.

When would you go about giving the feedback? It is suggested that feedback should be given at a time close to the event occurring. You will have to balance this decision with an evaluation of the suitability of the time available during a shift, at the end of the shift or at a pre-arranged time other than during the day of the shift. It depends on how busy you are and any other situational factors. However, do not let these factors obstruct you from your task. If this is the first time you are to give feedback you may want to let your ward manager know and practise how you are going to handle the situation with them. They can also give you support when the issue is raised in the team meeting.

Further reading

Grant, A and Goodman, B (2018) *Communication and Interpersonal Skills in Nursing* (4th edition). London: SAGE.

An accessible introduction to the subject.

Useful websites

www.nhsemployers.org/employershandbook/job-evaluation-handbook/job%20evaluation%20 handbook.pdf

Provides information on the Agenda for Change bands – see especially Chapters 5 and 6.

www.nhsemployers.org/PayAndContracts/AgendaForChange/KSF/Simplified-KSF/Pages/ SimplifiedKSF.aspx

Introduction to the NHS Knowledge and Skills Framework and its links to the NHS Agenda for Change National Pay Agreement.

http://rapidbi.com/created/personaldevelopmentplan.html#formonthejobdevelopmentrecord

Link to an example of a personal development plan from a commercial organisation.

http://revalidation.nmc.org.uk/welcome-to-revalidation

The NMC's webpages dedicated to the requirements for revalidation.

www.nmc.org.uk/about-us/our-role/who-we-regulate/nursing-associates/

The NMC's webpages about nursing associates.

www.qca.org.uk

Website of the Qualifications and Curriculum Authority.

www.nhsemployers.org/your-workforce/retain-and-improve/managing-your-workforce/ appraisals/appraisal-tools-and-tips

NHS Employers appraisal tools and tips.

Chapter 5 · Conflict management and negotiation skills

(Continued)

At the point of registration, the registered nurse will be able to:

3.10 demonstrate the skills and abilities required to recognise and assess people who show signs of self-harm and/or suicidal ideation.
3.11 undertake routine investigations, interpreting and sharing findings as appropriate.

Chapter aims

After reading this chapter, you will be able to:

- identify situations which may cause conflict;
- discuss strategies for preventing conflict;
- demonstrate awareness of methods of managing conflict;
- comment on your own ability to understand and manage yourself in difficult situations involving interpersonal conflict.

Introduction

Nursing involves caring for people during some of the most physically and emotionally difficult times of their lives. As well as patients, nurses meet relatives, friends and carers of patients, who may themselves be distressed and anxious. In some circumstances, nurses and other care staff can become upset or angry with patients, relatives, visitors or each other.

Within any clinical setting there is the potential for anxiety, confusion, distress, hurt and pain to erupt into conflict. Sometimes distress arises on account of a patient's physical, psychological or spiritual condition. At other times, frustration may surface because of apparent failures within systems, poor communication, lack of understanding or perceived or real rudeness.

Conflict may arise between patients and care staff; between patients; between care staff; between patients and significant others; or between staff and patients' significant others. Recognising the potential for conflict and learning how to prevent and manage conflict are all key skills in leadership and management. Perhaps the most important skill aspiring nurse leaders can have, however, is the ability to understand and manage themselves in such situations.

The purpose of this chapter is to enable you to explore some of the issues that contribute to the development of conflict in the clinical setting, and to examine strategies to prevent these occurring or to defuse such situations when they do occur.

What is conflict?

Understanding what conflict is and why it arises is fundamentally important in understanding both how to prevent it from occurring and how to manage it once it has arisen. Conflict is the expression of a disagreement between two or more parties that arises out of a difference in opinion, needs or desires. It is important to recognise that conflict is not usually about the individual; it is more likely to arise as a response to an individual's perception of a situation, behaviour or circumstance. The prevention of conflict, therefore, has as much, if not more, to do with the management of perception as with anything else.

Not all conflict is physical in nature, although what started as a disagreement, a heated discussion or an argument can soon escalate to violence if it is not handled well. The following example encourages you to think through an everyday situation in a hospital to increase your understanding of how easily a confrontational situation can develop.

Case study: The protracted wait

Stan is a busy man who attends hospital regularly for monitoring of his emphysema. The hospital is quite old, and Stan is forced to wait in the corridor along with the rest of the people attending the clinic because there is no waiting room. The corridor is cold and draughty and has a constant stream of people through it. Stan has waited over an hour past his allotted appointment time and is fed up, not only with the hanging around but with having to sit in the corridor. Stan approaches the receptionist and demands to know how much longer he will have to wait. The receptionist's response, while polite, is not helpful as she does not know why the appointments are running so far behind. Stan is upset by the lack of information he is given and the seemingly poor communication within the team. He shouts at the receptionist for being 'incompetent'.

This case study illustrates how perception and the physical environment can contribute to bad feeling. Stan is aggrieved at having to wait in an environment that is not designed for the purpose for which it is being used. He is forced to wait for a protracted period of time but does not know why. When Stan tries to find out why he is waiting, he does not get what he considers to be a reasonable response. The receptionist is not being rude, but Stan's perception of the fact she is unable to give him a reason for the delay is that his needs are not being met. He, perhaps reasonably, finds this unacceptable.

We can imagine the same scenario acted out in various ways which may lead to different outcomes. The receptionist might tell Stan to sit down and wait, thus escalating the situation to one of open conflict. She might apologise for the delay and say that she will find out what is happening and come back to him, thus meeting his need to feel that he is being taken seriously. She might empathise with Stan about his situation and say how bad it is for her as well; while this may distract Stan from shouting at her, it may lead to his anger being focused at other staff in the hospital. Evidently there may be little that she, or indeed many leaders or managers, can do about the physical surroundings (since this may require a considerable investment of money) but they can and must exercise control over the psychosocial, interpersonal environment of care. Caring enough to manage the psychosocial environment is a reflection of the values of respect for people and person-centredness and demonstrates the leader's compassion. Remember, leaders often set the vision for, and role model how, members of the team will behave.

What is also clear from this scenario is that the prevention of conflict is both everyone's business and in everyone's interests. It may seem to some that it is the role of managers, senior staff and security to deal with issues of conflict when they arise. What the protracted-wait scenario shows is that this perception is wrong. Being polite and appearing to be helpful is the role of all staff, whether they be care professionals, students or support workers. Clearly, and as is explored later in the chapter, one of the roles of the manager in this sort of scenario is to look for ways in which such situations can be managed better in the future to achieve better **outcomes** (that is, experiences of care) for patients.

Why managing conflict is important

The need to manage conflict effectively may seem obvious: conflict is just not nice. That said, it being not nice is only a small part of why conflict needs to be managed in care settings. There are many good reasons why managing conflict is important in the context of leadership and management, and these go beyond merely preventing an unpleasant situation.

The first reason that conflict management in care environments is important is that it can negatively affect the experiences of patients and clients (Kim et al., 2017). This applies equally to those involved in the conflict and those forced to witness it. The same is true of the staff in a department or team when conflict occurs regularly (McKibben, 2017). The negative experiences of staff will almost certainly affect their ability to care, and may give rise to absence through sickness associated with stress. Continued poor management of conflict may cause some staff to leave their posts, creating recruitment and retention issues, which has the potential to exacerbate local tensions and conflict.

Managing complaints and conflicts properly can lead to benefits for the team and the organisation. Recurrent complaints arising from the provision of care may be turned around to create opportunities for development. If conflict and complaints arise out of people's perceptions of the care they receive, then these can be used to help redesign both the ways in which care is delivered and the nature of the care itself. A key message for leaders and managers in the management of conflict is, therefore, about learning from it. Effectively managed, perhaps using **clinical supervision** (see Chapter 6) and the use of emotional intelligence techniques and individual reflection (McCloughen and Foster, 2018), conflict may prove to be a catalyst for innovation and creativity. **Total quality management** and good governance require nurse leaders and managers to recognise and engage in practices which improve both the processes and practices of healthcare; this includes responding to complaints, criticism and compliments from clients.

The best leaders, teams and organisations don't ignore adverse comments, they use them to redesign the delivery of care, thereby preventing issues from mounting up so that they become complaints. Teams that learn from their mistakes grow and develop and are often said to have a learning culture (see Chapter 8).

While there is no specific legislation in the UK covering workplace conflict or bullying, the Health and Safety at Work etc. Act (1974) makes it plain that employers have a duty of care for the health of their employees, and this includes their mental well-being. Legislation against discrimination on the grounds of age, sex, disability or ethnicity does exist, and requires that managers behave in an equitable manner toward all their employees, as required in the Equality Act (HM Government, 2010), and that they protect employees from harassment in the workplace. This requires managers, leaders and all care staff to be aware of situations that might lead to conflict, and to manage them and the behaviour of staff effectively.

Consider the following case study, where conflict arising out of the way in which a service is provided is reflected on and used to develop a better way of working, with potential to improve patients' experience.

Case study: The pain clinic

The pain clinic in the local district general hospital provides many services to local people, one of which is minor pain-relieving procedures requiring a short period of sedation. Each morning ten people are admitted to the clinic to undergo procedures such as facet joint injections and selective nerve root blocks. Each procedure is quite short but requires a small amount of sedation, so it usually takes about three hours to get through the whole procedures list.

Tom is asked to attend the clinic at 8 a.m. in order to have an injection to help manage his back pain. Tom duly arrives at 8 a.m. and sits in a waiting room, along with the other nine people. By 9.30 a.m. Tom is still waiting to be admitted as he is the last on the procedures list for that day. Tom is irritated by the wait as he is in pain and the chairs in the waiting area are uncomfortable. He asks Emma, the nurse admitting the patients, why he has been brought in so early when it is clear he will not need to be in a bed until about 11 a.m. Emma responds that it is just the way the clinic runs. Tom protests loudly that this is silly and that there has to be a better way of running things.

(Continued)

(Continued)

Another patient joins in, saying he feels as if they are being treated like cattle, being forced to wait for no apparent good reason. Both Tom and the other patient become quite excited and start to talk loudly about how ridiculous it all is, until they are both called in to be admitted.

Emma is quite intimidated by what has happened. She reflects that this is a regular occurrence and perhaps the patients have a point about the way in which the clinic is run. She decides to talk to Hamida, the clinical nurse manager, about the complaints at her next supervision.

Hamida points out that the orthopaedic day unit in the same hospital sends out different appointments for admissions on surgery days, with an hour between patients. The staggered admission times mean one nurse can comfortably admit and prepare three or four people for surgery on the same day and no one is kept waiting unnecessarily. Emma reflects on this and decides she should go and see what the orthopaedic unit are doing, to understand the pros and cons of their approach with a view to adopting the practice in the pain clinic.

What we can see in this case study is that patients have a real issue with being kept waiting, especially since they are in pain. Rather than ignoring this, hiding away or perhaps leaving the clinic, Emma takes on a leadership role and seeks to turn a problem into something that works for everyone's benefit. She uses reflection on the situation and then seeks help and support, in her supervision, from a more experienced member of the team. Any changes to the way the clinic is run are, then, a good example of the service being responsive to people's needs and an exercise in good governance.

Perhaps the second key message of managing potential conflict is to listen to what is being said, rather than just to how it is being said. As we can see, the patients in this scenario are making a valid point. A third lesson might be to seek help in understanding and solving potential issues, as Emma did.

Again, this case study shows the value of learning from and acting upon complaints, or adverse comments, to improve the quality of care provision. If we can do this, we demonstrate our engagement, both as nurses and as leaders, with improving the lives of our patients.

Identifying potential sources of conflict

Conflict is a constant possibility in any organisation where there are human interactions (Gerardi, 2015). The potential for conflict to arise in the hospital or other clinical setting is compounded by the type of work that occurs there (Kim et al., 2016). People visiting hospitals or other healthcare facilities, either as patients or visitors, are in physical and psychological distress. This means they are vulnerable, particularly if they do not understand what is happening. The fact that healthcare is often delivered in an autocratic manner also makes people feel vulnerable.

This vulnerability is perhaps not, in itself, something that nurses can eliminate. However, recognising it and doing something about it may make the difference between conflict arising or not. What is clear is that feeling vulnerable makes some people defensive and aggressive (Kim et al., 2016), and in identifying this, nurses, along with all care professionals, can do a lot to avert conflict.

Taking a leadership role in the management of conflict is every nurse's role. As we saw in Chapter 1 on the experience of leadership, this involves seeing the bigger picture and understanding how the structures within which we work affect both us and the people we work with. In good part these sentiments are reflected in the increasing importance of user consultation and patient involvement forums. Clearly, the best way to understand how care is experienced is to ask the people experiencing it and the best way to improve how care is experienced is, again, to involve those in receipt of care.

It is worth reflecting on the effect a lack of understanding can have on how we feel about ourselves and others around us, and how this lack of understanding can create a real sense of vulnerability.

Activity 5.1   Reflection

Think about your own experiences of care, or perhaps those of a family member. What are your enduring memories of the way care was delivered? Did you think at the time that things could have been done better? What was the communication like? Has your view on the delivery of care changed because of your experience of being a nurse? What is it about the delivery of care which has changed because of your increased understanding of nursing?

There are some possible answers and thoughts at the end of the chapter.

This activity emphasises that anxiety is a natural response to the unknown, and what people do and say can have a great impact. Understanding what may create feelings of vulnerability in ourselves can help us to understand which issues might create vulnerability in others. Managing our encounters with others, and recognising the potential for conflict that arises out of our interactions, allows us to demonstrate the important, people-centred aspects of leadership.

The potential for conflict can be heightened by the inequitable distribution of power within a team (Greer et al., 2017) (for more on managing conflict in teams, see Chapter 3). The manner in which we choose to present ourselves to others can heighten feelings of inadequacy and fear. The specialist knowledge we have in an area, and the position we hold, can be used to create barriers between us, our team and our patients. The idea of separation created by titles and roles is well demonstrated in the theories of **binary thinking** and **othering**, which demonstrate how we can create our own identities by comparing and contrasting ourselves with others (Davies, 2004).

We like to identify ourselves in various different ways as perhaps a parent, a partner, a nurse or a student. While these identities mean that we can explain who we are and what we do, they can also create a sense of difference between us and other people.

Concept summary: Binary thinking

Exploring the notion of binary identity and how this might apply in the clinical setting may help us to understand some of the ways in which conflict might arise. Within binary logic, 'A' is 'A' and anything that is not 'A' is 'something else'. Translated into the nursing workplace this may be seen as operating as: 'I am a nurse; you are not'; 'I know what is happening here; you do not'; 'I am the powerful professional; you are the compliant patient'; 'I know best; you do not'. You may have experienced this type of feeling yourself, perhaps as a student nurse, or in relation to another more 'powerful' professional.

In this sense, binary is seen as one of only two options, as in the code used to programme computers, where the only options available are 0 and 1. This tends to suggest strongly a sense of them and us – when someone is not one of us, they are something else.

In part, the differences expressed here represent some of the more negative aspects of creating for ourselves a professional identity which excludes others who do not share our identity (as a nurse, say) – sometimes called othering. This way of looking at ourselves creates a scheme whereby we see patients and non-nursing colleagues as 'other'. It is a small step from seeing ourselves as something different and set apart to the creation of conflict. Acting in ways that can be seen as highlighting and exploiting the differences between us as nurse and 'others' as patients, or us as leaders and 'others' as followers, runs counter to everything we identified as important in the way of exercising our common values in Chapter 1.

Conflict often arises because of perceived, if not real, differences between the needs, wants and desires of individuals. When we as nurses, and nurse leaders, remember that we are people first and nurses second, it will allow us to start to see something of the nature of the fear that being 'the other' brings. This realisation will help enable us not only to respond to, but to pre-empt, some of the conflict that arises as a result of fear and perceived isolation.

Activity 5.2   Critical thinking

Think about what binary thinking says about professional image and presentation of self to others in the care setting. How is binary identity used in the care setting to advantage the professional? Can you think of times someone has made you feel different or excluded by their behaviour? Have you used binary thinking to your own advantage? What approaches to self-presentation and leadership can stop these sorts of situations arising?

There are some possible answers and thoughts at the end of the chapter.

It is worth thinking critically about binary thinking here, not because it is a clever way of understanding how we create identities, but because it reflects a way in which conflict may be generated. Quite clearly, using binary thinking theory, we can see divisions between individuals are readily created when we start to see ourselves as something other than fellow human beings. This idea translates well into how we might think about preventing conflict, as well as how we lead others by example in the ways in which we interact with our managers, peers, those who work under our leadership and our patients.

Conflict may also arise in the clinical setting when staff disagree about the care and management of a particular patient. Sometimes conflict may arise because of an ethical dilemma, such as a family requesting that a loved one is not told her diagnosis when it appears she should be (Ellis, 2020). When ethical dilemmas occur, they can give rise to conflict between people with different views about how the issue should be resolved. Differences of views may then arise along professional boundaries, or between professionals and patients. Alternatively, they may result as a consequence of age, gender, personality traits, status, culture, religion or experience (Kim et al., 2017).

Binary theory helps us to understand what is going on in such situations where conflict arises. People who disagree with our point of view, instead of being accepted as people with another viewpoint, are regarded as 'other' and therefore become a legitimate target of attack. The role of the leader or manager in such situations is to focus the discussions back to the issue under dispute and away from the personalities involved.

The Chartered Institute of Personnel and Development (CIPD, 2021) identified general behaviour, disputes about performance, attendance at work and relationships between colleagues as being the main causes of conflict at work. Of note, the CIPD (2021) identify what they call less obvious causes of conflict to include talking over people, not valuing others' opinions, ignoring people and poor personal hygiene.

Bullying takes many forms in the healthcare sector and can involve staff bullying other staff, staff bullying patients, patients bullying staff and visitors and relatives bullying staff. In a survey of NHS staff in England, around 19 per cent reported having been bullied, harassed or abused in the last year by other NHS staff (NHS Survey Coordination Centre, 2021) with about 45 per cent of NHS employees claiming relationships at work are strained. Despite 2020 being an unusual year as the COVID-19 pandemic affected the NHS, these figures are, sadly, not all that unusual.

Bullying can take many forms. Some bullying is deliberate, whereas other bullying arises out of differences in perception and poor communication. Gossiping about someone, spreading rumours, ridiculing someone, as well as being consistently rude or abusive, all constitute bullying behaviour.

Case study: Bullying

Steve was a newly qualified nurse who prior to becoming a nurse had undertaken a first degree and Master's degree in biology. Steve joined the team in the intensive care unit at his local hospital as a junior staff nurse and greatly enjoyed his job.

Amanda was one of the unit sisters who had been qualified for many years and was a very experienced nurse. When Steve was on shift with Amanda he was often allocated the patient in the isolation room. Steve got the feeling that Amanda did not like him and noticed that he was often overlooked for breaks and was never allowed to look after unusual cases in the main unit when she was on duty.

Steve felt that he was being bullied and started to become very unhappy at work. Steve raised his concerns with one of the unit charge nurses, Des. Des had also noticed the behaviours that Steve described and advised Steve to have a word with Amanda about it. When Steve asked to talk to Amanda, she was dismissive, but Steve persisted. In the office Steve raised his concerns, saying he had joined the team to learn how to nurse in the intensive therapy unit and he was keen to be useful. He said he felt excluded by Amanda and that she appeared to have taken a dislike to him for no apparent reason. Amanda started to cry.

Amanda admitted that she felt intimidated by Steve as she had found out he had two degrees and she did not even have a diploma. Amanda admitted she was worried about her position in the team with bright young things threatening her status.

In this real-life case study, we can see that Amanda's behaviour has arisen out of her own fears about her position in the team. It could have all been so different, however; she might have treated Steve in the manner she did because she did not like men, because he was gay, because he was from a different ethnic background or because she did not like his religious views. Quite clearly, any one of these alternative explanations is unacceptable, as is the fact that she was using her position to bully him because she felt threatened. What is also important about this scenario is that Steve could quite easily have thought he was being bullied because of a personal characteristic, and escalated the issue to management, making a bad situation worse.

As well as understanding that bullying can take many forms, the other message from this scenario is that leaders and managers need also to be careful that their actions are not misinterpreted as bullying. This requires, as we have discussed before, that the manager knows their staff group well and acts to develop a positive workplace culture.

Activity 5.3   Evidence-based practice and research

Unfortunately, bullying and harassment are common workplace occurrences (see the statistic cited earlier). When you are next at work, find a copy of the local bullying and harassment policy and familiarise yourself with the definitions it contains, as well as the local practices in relation to it. Also, look on the internet and find some definitions of bullying and list some of the effects it can have on an individual experiencing it. It is worth looking at the NHS staff survey site identified in useful websites at the end of this chapter, as some of the statistics make salutary reading.

As the answers to this activity will depend on the policy available in your own workplace, no outline answer is given.

What all the examples of how conflict could emerge in the clinical setting have in common is that they all come about as a result of communication issues. Handling communication, perception, relationships and being self-aware are, therefore, important elements of conflict prevention and management.

Managing to reduce the potential for conflict

What we have seen so far in this chapter points to the fact that much conflict can be avoided. From the leadership and management perspective, as well as from the perspective of individual behaviours, there are a number of strategies that can be used to help prevent conflict. The key to reducing the potential for conflict lies in managing the environment of care in such a way that it is focused on achieving high-quality patient outcomes. Key among the strategies for conflict prevention and resolution are using experienced staff, engendering a spirit of collaboration, problem-solving and integrated management styles (Lahana et al., 2019).

There is good reason to think, as a leader or manager, that treating the staff in our team as people first and as staff second can lead to an increase in the level of trust and reduce the potential for conflict – as well as signposting the values we want the staff to display in their interactions with each other and patients. Leaders who show their values by adopting a servant leadership style of management engender trust in their teams, and with trust comes a culture which is more open and honest, and which reduces conflict (Setyaningrum et al., 2020).

In his widely cited piece of work, Scholtes (1998) identifies two elements to the generation of trust in leaders: first, that leaders are competent and able to do their job, and second, they demonstrate that they care for the staff who work with them (see also p46). It is in the demonstration of caring about the welfare of staff, the exercise of the value of *person-centredness*, that the leader sets the tone for how the team will work with each other and patients.

The strategies for managing to reduce the potential for conflict are, like so many issues and ideas in leadership and management, heavily interlinked. The culture of the organisation, department or team all contribute to the ways in which conflict arises, is prevented, recognised and dealt with. Creating a culture where we learn from our mistakes, and environments that allow people to develop and grow as individuals and professionals, will have a great impact on reducing the likelihood of conflict arising in a team. While **learning organisations** are explored in more depth in Chapter 8, it is worth noting here that an organisation that allows people to make mistakes, learn from their mistakes and develop, is more likely to reduce the likelihood of conflict arising, and to handle conflict in a meaningful way. The same message translates well down to team level, where a manager who encourages and supports learning enables members of the team to understand the root causes of conflict and how to deal with them.

Managing situations where conflict arises

When conflict does arise, there are a number of approaches that can be taken to manage it. The choice of which approaches to use will depend on the nature of the conflict: who is involved, where it is taking place and whether the conflict is physical or purely verbal in nature. The choice of approach to managing the situation will also make a great deal of difference to the potential outcome of the situation. Thought should always be given to what strategy is right in any given situation, but if this is not possible it is always best to start with the minimum intervention required and scale up.

Table 5.1 gives some often cited ideas about general approaches to managing conflict, along with when to use them and their pros and cons.

What seems clear from the strategies in Table 5.1 is that different approaches will suit different scenarios. Constant use of one strategy will lead people to thinking that you do not have the **emotional intelligence** to work out when to change what you do in response to different situations. Knowing what strategy to employ is not something that is easily taught; like emotional intelligence, it is something that comes with time, experience and reflection.

Junior staff often use dodging, because they do not have the experience to draw on which tells them which strategy to use in managing conflict. As identified earlier, the use of supervision and reflection are important in learning from conflict situations and developing a bank of experience and emotional intelligence techniques for managing future conflict.

Collaboration: creates a potential situation where everyone can win, and allows for creative solutions. It requires that the situation is worked through and a solution found which addresses concerns. This is useful where the conflict arises between individuals who either trust each other a lot or where there is pre-existing enmity. Collaboration, while it may be an effective means of managing conflict, can be time consuming and is open to abuse if both parties are not really committed to it.

Compromising: leads to a situation where everyone involved has to give a little ground. This may prove beneficial where the parties in the dispute are equally committed to their own point of view and where they are of similar status. It can speed up the process of resolving a dispute, but only when the exact outcome is not too important. Compromise may lead to a solution that is not acceptable to anyone, and may not work if the sides are too far apart at the start.

Accommodating: is useful when one side of a conflict realises the issue is more important to the other side, or that they are wrong. Accommodating allows for **social capital** to be built up and called upon later, and helps to maintain relationships which may be more important than the disagreement. The problem with being accommodating is that people may see it as a sign of weakness and take advantage.

Competing: sometimes other avenues of reaching agreement have been exhausted, so when the point being made is correct, it is important not to give in easily. On other occasions, when someone is trying to forcibly get his or her way it is best to challenge the person. The experienced leader or manager will recognise that competition can escalate some conflicts and it may not be wise when the conflict is, or may become, physical in nature.

Dodging: is perhaps the best strategy when the conflict is not important, you are too busy to deal with an issue at that time, you need to cool off or there is no chance of winning. Dodging the issue can, however, make matters worse in the long run and may allow a transgressor to win. Dodging can be used as a short-term strategy by the manager but rarely results in a satisfactory solution to the issue of conflict.

Table 5.1   General approaches to managing conflict situations

Source: Adapted from Thomas and Kilmann (1974).

Activity 5.4   Critical thinking

Sue has been admitted to the orthopaedic ward following a fall in which she broke her arm. It is late evening and, just as visiting is about to finish, Dave, Sue's husband, arrives to visit her. You are asked by the ward sister to tell Dave that he must leave in five minutes, despite him having just arrived. Dutifully you tell Dave that visiting is nearly over and he must leave. Dave is angered by this and aggressively states that he has only just been able to get there and he should be allowed to see his wife and that the rules are ridiculous.

Use the strategies identified in Table 5.1 to think about the alternative approaches you might use to handle this situation. Which approach(es) best fit this particular scenario? Why?

There are some possible answers and thoughts at the end of the chapter.

This activity, drawn from a real-life experience, demonstrates how rigid adherence to rules can be construed as insensitivity and so inflame what must already be a worrying situation. Clearly, the right approach would have been not to provoke conflict in the first place, but to ask whether Dave knew the visiting times and why he had been so late.

Perhaps a compromise might then have been reached without the need for generating bad feeling. Always the number one rule of conflict management is to avoid starting it in the first place.

There is a key message for the novice manager – rules need to be interpreted within the context of individual situations and not followed blindly. The emotionally intelligent manager will realise that on occasions breaking the rules is the right thing to do, and that in exercising wise choices such as this they are demonstrating leadership rather than being weak.

Negotiation

Although it is easy to imagine **negotiation** is the starting point for dealing with all conflicts, in some instances it is not. Negotiation means trying to reach an agreement with another party when both parties share the same overall objective but perhaps differ on how this objective might be achieved. Negotiating is the process that is undertaken in order to reach a compromise solution to an issue. One of the fringe benefits of successful negotiation is that the relationship that builds up in a successful negotiation may lead to future collaboration.

The first rule of negotiation is to know what it is you want to achieve – the outcome that is acceptable to you. Once you know what is acceptable as a solution you know what ground you can give in the process and what you need to defend to achieve your goal. This is also the time to decide what the points of conflict are: why do you and the other party not agree?

The second most important negotiating skill is listening (Abdelhafez and Hossny, 2019). Listening not only allows you to understand the other person's point of view; it also creates opportunity for you to ask sensible questions about what they are saying.

The third rule of negotiation is to build on small successes, get agreement on small issues and then work up toward the main issue of the conflict. This allows for an environment of collaboration and agreement to be created and built upon. What are you willing to give up, and what is the other party willing to give up as part of the process?

The ability to negotiate will depend on many factors, including biases and emotions, while the local culture, including power relationships and perceived status of the individual involved, may make it a difficult strategy to pursue (Brett and Thompson, 2016).

Activity 5.5   Reflection

Taking the idea that negotiation, like most approaches to conflict resolution, requires **active listening**, consider the ways in which you can demonstrate to someone that you are listening to them. Consider your body language, the non-verbal and verbal cues you can give them and the sorts of questions you might ask to demonstrate engagement. Think especially about a recent interaction you have had which could have been tricky had you not used your verbal and non-verbal skills and, as with all reflection, think about what you did well and what you might do next time you encounter a similar situation.

As the answer to this activity is based on your own reflection, there is no specimen answer at the end of the chapter.

Mediation

Sometimes a dispute or conflict between individuals cannot be resolved by the individuals themselves. At this stage there is a need for a third party to help find a resolution to the issue. One approach to conflict resolution is the use of **mediation** (Lahana et al., 2019). Mediation is not about the settlement of a dispute by the imposition of an agreement; rather, it is a means of facilitating a resolution that both parties can agree to. A mediator's role is that of an impartial third party who helps progress a solution to a problem.

In mediation, the mediator listens to both sides of an issue, sometimes in private, and then brings the two sides together to discuss their grievances. The mediator will try to identify common ground, things the two parties can agree on, and uses these to start building a resolution to a problem. Fundamental to the process of mediation is that both sides in a dispute agree to take part in the mediation process and are willing to seek agreement. Reaching agreement is not simply about compromise, or one side backing down; instead, mediation seeks to build on small agreements until a consensus is reached.

Mediation is especially useful where two sides have a history of not working together, as it helps to build relationships which allow for future development and joint working. For a leader, this may mean facilitating discussions between two members of a team who do not get on, or who are in conflict about some aspect of their working life.

Activity 5.6   Evidence-based practice and research

Next time you are in the workplace, take the time to find the human resources policy which covers conflict between individuals and read the section about mediation. Also, using the link at the end of this chapter, go online and look at the Advisory, Conciliation and Arbitration Service's description of mediation.

As the answer to this activity is based on what you find, there is no specimen answer at the end of the chapter.

Arbitration

When the processes of negotiation or mediation fail, it may become necessary to look for other ways of resolving a dispute between two parties. Arbitration and conciliation, like mediation, employ the services of a third, impartial individual to help reach a resolution.

In arbitration, the role of the third party is to decide on and impose a final solution to the conflict. The decision that is reached is based on the third party gathering together all of the facts and coming to some conclusion about what should be done to resolve the issue. An arbitrator has the authority to impose the decision on those in dispute. However, there may be instances when one or both sides in a dispute feel unhappy about the result, creating continued tensions in the workplace. Leaders who have to arbitrate will, therefore, need to stick to their values and demonstrate emotional intelligence in managing such situations.

Case study: The rota

Ann and Claire are junior staff nurses on the same ward. There is a concert by a well-known band in the town in a couple of weekends' time and both Ann and Claire want to go. Both nurses are rostered to be at work at the time of the concert and so both approach the ward sister and ask for an early shift or the day off instead. The sister says that she needs one of them to work and that they must sort it out between them.

Ann and Claire, who aren't the best of friends anyway, soon get into a verbal fight about who should have the opportunity to go to the concert. The argument spills over from the staff room to the ward and the sister has to take them both into her office. Both Ann and Claire claim they need to have the evening off more, and again begin to squabble. The sister has to intervene and suggests that she will have to make the decision and they will have to abide by it as that is what is required. Reluctantly they both agree. The sister says that, as she cannot choose between them, then the original rota which was written without any knowledge of the concert must stand.

Whistle blowing

So far, the examples we have used all have some reasonable explanation and resolving the issues they create is relatively easy. Sadly, this is not always the case. Sometimes, there are situations of conflict, bullying or harassment which are not amenable to being dealt with locally. When the culture of a workplace is such that the manager will not address issues of poor practice or bullying, then sometimes the only ethically right thing left to do is whistle blow (Ion et al., 2016). Whistle blowing offers one avenue for people who witness, or who are experiencing, conflict or bullying in the workplace to get help.

Essentially, whistle blowing is the act of bringing an important issue to the attention of someone in authority. Sometimes whistle blowing occurs within a team or organisation. If there are issues with an organisation, however, whistle blowing may need to be external. Within the NHS there are policies in place for both forms of whistle blowing. In certain circumstances, these allow the whistle blower to remain anonymous.

The Public Information Disclosures Act 1998 (HM Government, 1998) protects people who blow the whistle about poor practices specifically where the worker has real concerns about any one of a number of issues. Such issues for the manager or leader may include the health and safety of workers (Health and Safety Executive, n.d.). As discussed earlier, this includes protecting staff from abuse and conflict and the subsequent impact of this on their health.

Activity 5.7   Evidence-based practice and research

Using the useful websites at the end of the chapter, look up the Public Interest Disclosure Act 1998 and the Health and Safety at Work etc. Act 1974, and consider how these apply to where you work as well as where you study.

As the answer to this activity is based on what you find, there is no specimen answer at the end of the chapter.

Deciding to blow the whistle is a big step for anyone involved in conflict or bullying. In all such situations it is better, if possible, to try to come to some solution more locally. However, there are times, perhaps involving a legal or ethical issue, where whistle blowing may be the right thing to do. One example can be found within the key findings of the Francis report (2013), which demonstrated too great a degree of tolerance of poor standards and of risk to patients, along with assumptions that monitoring, performance management or intervention was the responsibility of someone else.

These key findings suggest the culture prevented good practice in both care and in the communication of the lack of good care. Good care and intolerance of poor standards and risk to patients is everyone's concern and the need to do something about it, potentially by blowing the whistle, is something all nurse leaders should encourage.

Managing yourself

It may seem strange to say this toward the end of a chapter dealing with conflict, but the first point of reference for anyone involved in conflict is to ask if they, themselves, are the problem. Management of yourself and your relationships with other people is an important step on the road to becoming an effective leader and manager of others. Who wants to be led by a person who cannot manage themselves?

If you are not sure if you are the cause of the conflict you are experiencing, there are two things you can do to be certain you are not. First, ask yourself the question, 'do I have a problem with a lot of the people I work with?' If the answer is yes, then you may well be the person who has the problem, if no then you might not be. Second, ask people you trust, perhaps people who are not dependent on you, if they think you are the cause of conflict. Again if they say yes, you are probably the problem; if they say no, you may not be.

Since differences of opinion, perception and power all play a role in creating conflict situations, it is important for prospective leaders and managers to be aware of the influences on their thinking as well as how they come across to others. It may be tempting to think that this can be achieved purely through reflection, but reflection alone is likely to produce a flawed view. Self-management is as much about self-development as it is about being aware of your own opinions, and if you are to develop you need to take on board feedback from other individuals.

It would be easy to say that, in order to avoid unnecessary conflict, you should always follow what you believe to be the moral and ethical thing to do. This oversimplifies the case for self-management, however. Evidently there are some ethical and moral principles which, if you believe in them and act on them, will mean you can usually justify your actions – it is the exercise of the principles that allows others to see the sorts of values we hold dear and what sort of person we therefore are (Ellis, 2020). Such principles might include treating others as equals and always trying to be fair. Rigid adherence to rules, as we saw in Activity 4.4, can lead to problems, and so part of managing yourself is to learn when to adapt what you do to the situation. This means being open to the views of others and being able to adapt your behaviours when necessary, while not abandoning important ethical principles.

In essence this is about good communication, awareness of how others see you and how you behave, and being aware of the perceptions of others. Mayer and Salovey (1993, p433) termed this ability 'emotional intelligence' and described it as *a type of social intelligence that involves the ability to monitor one's own and others' emotions, to discriminate among them, and to use the information to guide one's thinking and actions*. There are essentially four elements to the Mayer–Salovey model of emotional intelligence: (1) the ability to identify emotions in yourself and others; (2) the ability to use emotion to communicate; (3) the ability to understand how emotional information is used to construct meaning; and (4) the ability to manage your own emotions.

Being able to read and understand the emotions that lie behind your own behaviours and the behaviours of others is helpful in identifying whether conflict is a result of your behaviours or a reasonable response to the behaviours of others. To grow your emotional intelligence, it is important to reflect on your own motivations, to ask others about their motivations, and to put this in the context of the situation in which you find yourself. The essence of conflict management, therefore, is honest communication with yourself and with others.

Chapter summary

In this chapter we have identified some of the causes of conflict which arise in the clinical setting. We have identified that perception plays a large part in how people feel about a situation, and that poor management of a situation, frequently the result of poor or non-existent communication, is often the root cause of conflict.

We have identified that there are a number of strategies that can be employed by the nurse leader to prevent conflict from arising, to identify situations in which conflict may arise and to manage conflict when it does occur. The fundamental messages for the management of conflict appear to lie in the need for good communication, management of self, and treating others as equals.

We have seen that not all conflict can be dealt with by the individuals involved in the conflict, and that it is sometimes necessary to involve a third party, either to help those in conflict come to a negotiated settlement or to have a settlement imposed. As with all aspects of nursing and interpersonal relationships, the key skill of reflection (both alone and with others) is helpful in resolving situations that arise.

Activities: Brief outline answers

Activity 5.1 Reflection (p95)

Being on the receiving end of care can be an enlightening experience for health and social care professionals. The priorities we have when we are nursing often change dramatically when we are the ones being nursed. As a nurse you might prioritise getting the drug round done, but as a patient you might prioritise getting pain relief when you want it. As a nurse you might prioritise doing a dressing, but as a patient you might prioritise getting an explanation of your care.

It is easy to see how conflicting priorities can lead to misunderstandings and conflict. Nurses might think they are doing well in getting the drug round done, but if you are the patient at the end of the round you might think that your needs are being overlooked and that the nurse is being callous. Taking the patient's view of what they are experiencing can be enlightening for nurses and help them understand the causes of conflict in situations where they had previously considered the patient to be being difficult or unreasonable.

Activity 5.2 Critical thinking (p96)

The answers to this issue lie in the way in which we choose to present ourselves to others, as well as the values we hold and the ways in which we choose to express these values. If we are quite clear in our interactions with patients and more junior staff that we are the knowledgeable professional and they are not, we will cause antagonism. If we choose to remember, as nurses and leaders of people, that we too are people and that we are dealing with people, then the ways in which we interact will demonstrate this, and will be less likely to give rise to behaviours that cause conflict to occur.

Avoiding othering is in fact quite simple. Treating people as equals, asking their permission to do things – 'May I take your blood pressure please?' and 'Would you please take Mrs Smith to the toilet?' – demonstrate that we value the people we are interacting with, rather than treating them as in some way inferior.

Activity 5.4 Critical thinking (p101)

- Collaboration will require a discussion to take place about Dave's concerns and that you show understanding in reaching a solution that addresses them.
- Compromising will allow you to reach a mutually agreeable solution with Dave – perhaps allowing him to stay a little longer, but only on this occasion.
- Accommodating: allowing Dave to stay because of the circumstances would perhaps seem reasonable and will defuse the situation, but it may mean he abuses the system in the future.
- Competing would mean demanding Dave leaves and perhaps calling security. This would alienate both Dave and Sue, and may not be a good idea in the long run.
- Dodging: just walking away and hoping Dave will leave is not really an option as other patients in the ward will see what has happened and may choose to do the same with their visitors or may be disturbed by Dave's continued presence.

Further reading

Codier, E (2020) *Emotional Intelligence in Nursing: Essentials for Leadership and Practice Improvement.* New York: Springer Publishing Company.

A book on emotional intelligence especially for nurses.

Grant, A and Goodman, B (2018) *Communication and Interpersonal Skills in Nursing* (4th edition). London: SAGE.

See especially Chapter 4 on understanding potential barriers to safe and effective practice.

Useful websites

www.cipd.co.uk/podcasts/shifting-perception-conflict

A podcast from the CIPD, on workplace conflict.

www.acas.org.uk/index.aspx?articleid=1364

The Advisory, Conciliation and Arbitration Service's guide to managing conflict at work.

www.acas.org.uk/index.aspx?articleid=1680

The Advisory, Conciliation and Arbitration Service's guide to mediation.

www.alchemyformanagers.co.uk/topics/G9Xf32ZuXQ4jL2YN.html

Alchemy for managers: a good overview of whistle blowing and the Public Interest Disclosure Act 1998.

www.hse.gov.uk/legislation/hswa.htm

The Health and Safety Executive's pages about the Health and Safety Act

www.nhsstaffsurveyresults.com/

The home of the NHS staff survey results and well worth a read.

www.nmc.org.uk/standards/guidance/raising-concerns-guidance-for-nurses-and-midwives/

The NMC's guidance on raising concerns and whistle blowing.

www.gov.uk/whistleblowing

UK governmental whistle blowing guidance.

www.danielgoleman.info/topics/emotional-intelligence

The website of the most widely cited writer on emotional intelligence.

Chapter 6   Coaching, mentoring and clinical supervision

NMC Standards of Proficiency for Registered Nurses

This chapter will address the following platforms and proficiencies:

Platform 1: Being an accountable professional

Registered nurses act in the best interests of people, putting them first and providing nursing care that is person-centred, safe and compassionate. They act professionally at all times and use their knowledge and experience to make evidence-based decisions about care. They communicate effectively, are role models for others, and are accountable for their actions. Registered nurses continually reflect on their practice and keep abreast of new and emerging developments in nursing, health and care.

At the point of registration, the registered nurse will be able to:

1.1   understand and act in accordance with the Code (2018): Professional standards of practice and behaviour for nurses, midwives and nursing associates, and fulfil all registration requirements.

1.11   communicate effectively using a range of skills and strategies with colleagues and people at all stages of life and with a range of mental, physical, cognitive and behavioural health challenges.

1.13   demonstrate the skills and abilities required to develop, manage and maintain appropriate relationships with people, their families, carers and colleagues.

1.14   provide and promote non-discriminatory, person-centred and sensitive care at all times, reflecting on people's values and beliefs, diverse backgrounds, cultural characteristics, language requirements, needs and preferences, taking account of any need for adjustments.

(Continued)

(Continued)

Platform 3: Assessing needs and planning care

Registered nurses prioritise the needs of people when assessing and reviewing their mental, physical, cognitive, behavioural, social and spiritual needs. They use information obtained during assessments to identify the priorities and requirements for person-centred and evidence-based nursing interventions and support. They work in partnership with people to develop person-centred care plans that take into account their circumstances, characteristics and preferences.

At the point of registration, the registered nurse will be able to:

3.4   understand and apply a person-centred approach to nursing care, demonstrating shared assessment, planning, decision making and goal setting when working with people, their families, communities and populations of all ages.

Platform 5: Leading and managing nursing care and working in teams

Registered nurses provide leadership by acting as a role model for best practice in the delivery of nursing care. They are responsible for managing nursing care and are accountable for the appropriate delegation and supervision of care provided by others in the team, including lay carers. They play an active and equal role in the interdisciplinary team, collaborating and communicating effectively with a range of colleagues.

At the point of registration, the registered nurse will be able to:

5.7   demonstrate the ability to monitor and evaluate the quality of care delivered by others in the team and lay carers.

5.8   support and supervise students in the delivery of nursing care, promoting reflection and providing constructive feedback, and evaluating and documenting their performance.

5.9   demonstrate the ability to challenge and provide constructive feedback about care delivered by others in the team, and support them to identify and agree individual learning needs.

5.10   contribute to supervision and team reflection activities to promote improvements in practice and services.

Chapter aims

After reading this chapter, you will be able to:

* identify different methods of coaching;
* describe the different approaches to practice supervision and assessment;
* understand the benefits of clinical supervision;
* recognise the signs of burnout and methods to reduce these effects.

Introduction

The main emphasis in this chapter is on the support of staff through leadership and management techniques such as coaching, mentoring and clinical supervision. This chapter will identify some of the different scenarios in which the leader or manager will undertake coaching, mentoring or supervision with team members. We will also consider various approaches to coaching, mentoring and supervision and discuss their respective pros and cons. In this chapter, we take the view that coaching, mentoring and supervision are all supportive and developmental functions of leadership, rather than seeing them as punitive. Because they are all regarded as developmental, coaching, mentoring and supervision contribute to the creation and maintenance of what is called a **learning culture**.

Because workplace environments, or cultures, are so important in protecting the well-being of staff, we will consider the causes and effects of staff burnout and what the leader or manager might do to promote a positive work–life balance culture which supports staff.

You may feel support and development are not the remit of the nurse leader, perhaps fitting better within the development team or at university but, in reality, the techniques and ideas contained within this chapter can be applied throughout the working day as the nurse leader encounters different situations at work. For example, mentoring or coaching techniques can quite easily be seen in action as the nurse provides direction and support to more junior staff who are providing care, while clinical supervision can happen informally when the team need to debrief following a difficult day at work. In any case, it is the reality of what happens in the patient-facing areas which matters and not the theory; this is where true clinical leadership is seen.

Coaching to improve performance

The term 'coaching' is more often used in the UK when referring to the training of athletes or performers and may be caricatured by a person with a whistle and clipboard. You do not need to be a coach to provide coaching, but you do need to understand some of the necessary skills and have an understanding of the general approach.

Increasingly the term coaching is seen as referring to an approach used in encouraging the development and application of workplace skills. Coaching in this sense is based upon the relationship between a manager or team leader and a team member; but might equally apply between a team leader and a member of their team, or between a registered nurse and a nursing associate.

In Chapter 4, we considered staff development and touched on performance appraisal and personal development planning as means of preparing and supporting staff to improve their knowledge and skills. Coaching is one method of supporting others to improve in an individually tailored manner. It is based upon a belief that individuals can develop skills and knowledge through frequent interactions (often called one-to-one meetings, 1:1s or, perhaps confusingly, supervisions) that are planned and carried out with an agreed outcome in mind.

The notion of coaching in organisations, and mentoring, which we will look at later in the chapter, as management tools began with the introduction of the people management and development literature. It can be traced back to the situational leadership model developed by Hersey and Blanchard in the 1960s (Hersey et al., 2007). The model is composed of four quadrants (Figure 6.1). Within their model, Hersey and Blanchard use the term coaching to mean the process by which the leader both leads and persuades followers to adopt a solution to a given situation. In this way the member(s) of staff is/are included both in the decision-making and in making suggestions toward the completion of the task. It is an approach that both motivates and builds team members' competence.

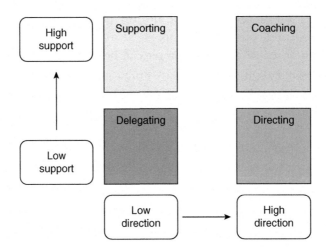

Figure 6.1 Hersey and Blanchard's situational leadership model (adapted)

Source: Adapted from Hersey et al. (2007).

In Chapter 4, we explored the work of Kotter (1990), who recognised the importance of matching one's leadership style to the level of commitment and competence of the individual staff member. Kotter's approach identifies to the manager when and how tasks should be passed on to the team member. This enables a leader to draw out the best in team members and identify where development needs to take place. The Hersey and Blanchard model extends this approach and stresses that the leader must be flexible and have at the forefront the developmental needs of the individual and not only the appropriate delegation method.

The leader needs to select an approach, or combination of approaches, from one of four leadership styles:

1. telling/directing;
2. selling/coaching;
3. participating/supporting;
4. delegating.

These are matched, respectively, with one of four follower styles, or developmental levels of maturity in the individual:

1. low competence/high commitment;
2. some competence/low commitment;
3. high competence/variable commitment;
4. high competence/high commitment.

Depending on the work maturity of the person, the leader provides high to low support along an axis of low to high direction. For example, the person with high commitment/high competence requires the least support and direction and can assume delegated tasks with minimal interference from the leader (as can be seen in Figure 6.1).

Case study: Teaching a procedure

David is a band 6 staff nurse, and Jasmine a new nursing associate. On Jasmine's second day, David spends 30 minutes telling her how to carry out a procedure to clean and redress a wound, with the expectation that she will do this herself once the knowledge and skills required for the task have been thoroughly explained. David gives Jasmine instructions on what to use, why, when, where and to whom. Then he tells her he will come back in two hours to see how she is getting on.

When David returns, the wound has not been dressed with the appropriate dressing and he has to redo it. This causes unnecessary discomfort to the patient and wastes time.

Although David may feel frustrated about this, questions have to be asked about the process of instruction that took place and whether it can be improved. Hersey and Blanchard maintain that leaders have to match the style of leadership to the maturity (or developmental style) and readiness (i.e. competence and motivation) of the person or team they are leading to perform a task. Thus, a simple telling and instruction session will not be sufficient. There needs to be an

(Continued)

(Continued)

assessment of the individual's learning style, level of comprehension, confidence and motivation, and a relationship needs to be established or developed between the leader and the 'follower'.

This means that David, as the senior, might be advised to take the following steps:

1. Make an overall assessment of Jasmine's scope of current tasks and activities. Determine her current workload and how she is coping with it.
2. Assess Jasmine's development level on the requested task by questioning and/or demonstration.
3. Decide on the leadership style.
4. Discuss with Jasmine the approach to be taken.
5. Follow up and discuss progress; correct where necessary.

Activity 6.1   Reflection

Think about when you have been working with a more junior member of staff and had to delegate a task to them. How did you do it and what steps did you take to explain what they needed to do? What factors did you consider? Did you consider their learning style? If you were to say which leadership approach you took, which one would it be? Knowing what you know now, what would you change next time you have to delegate?

You may find it helpful to revise your knowledge of Honey and Mumford's (2006) learning styles to help you consider how individuals learn. A web link is in the useful websites section at the end of the chapter to help you here.

As this answer is based on your own reflection, there is no outline answer at the end of the chapter.

Since the introduction of situational leadership, other approaches have been developed in coaching methods for work improvement. In the UK, the notion of coaching as a metaphor for improving performance came to prominence with the publication of *The Inner Game of Tennis* (1974), by Tim Gallwey, who went on to publish *The Inner Game of Work* (2000). The latter drew on a philosophy summarised as *Performance = Potential minus Interference*. Thus, the coach's job was to release the self-knowledge and potential that everyone possesses, rather than deliberately instructing an individual toward achievements. The key ingredient was to develop greater self-awareness and a sense of responsibility in the performer. This approach has subsequently crossed over into clinical practice, where the methods are frequently used to empower patients to develop self-efficacy in the management of chronic illnesses (Perlman and Abu Dabrh, 2020).

The GROW technique

Developed by Whitmore (1992) from the original Gallwey texts is a coaching technique that relies on using questions and which follows a structure to involve the person in problem solving as well as learning. Known as the GROW technique, the idea is to use a simple guided set of questions that can form the basis of a discussion in a coaching session or as a means of establishing the developmental level of a person to be supported. The aim is to assist the person to think about the problem/task at hand and identify a solution or range of options.

An easy way to remember the structure of the questions is to refer to the mnemonic that summarises the GROW technique in this way:

* Establish the *goal*.
* Examine the *reality*.
* Consider all *options*.
* Confirm the *will* to act.

This approach is helpful in improving motivation in people with basic knowledge, expertise and enthusiasm in a particular area. However, with inexperienced learners, applying GROW can be time consuming and not practical for day-to-day work-based situations (Parsloe and Leedham, 2009). For this approach to be effective, the questions need to be expanded, undertaken over a period of time and yet remain focused on the main goal to be achieved. The prominent factor is that the coaching is undertaken as a conversation, with two-way communication between the person and the leader or manager.

The 3 D technique

A more rapid approach is known as the 3 D technique. When time is really short and a solution to a problem has to be identified quickly, the technique is to identify elements on three dimensions:

1. The situation – for example timescales, lack of resources, lack of expertise.

2. People involved – for example, unhappy, impatient, unreliable, over-confident.

3. You – for example, lack of knowledge, conflicting priorities, general attitude.

From this analysis it is possible, by using questioning techniques around the dimensions, to draw out potential actions or plans.

Activity 6.3   Reflection

This activity is designed to help you with rapid coaching and skill building.

Practise the 3 D technique on yourself to coach yourself through a problem by following these six steps:

1. Define a current problem in a single sentence.
2. List three general issues relating to the problem situation.
3. List three issues relating to the people involved.
4. List three issues that relate specifically to you and the problem.
5. Choose one issue from each of your three lists of three issues.
6. Now identify one or more actions/options that are most likely to make progress in solving the problem.

As you are going through the steps, imagine you are asking yourself questions and make a note of the coaching questions you ask, so you can reflect later on whether they were the right questions to ask.

You may want to gain further skills in this approach by working with a fellow student or friend on a problem either you or they wish to solve. In this way you not only develop your own skills; you can also ask for feedback on the different types of questions you need to ask to elicit answers that are helpful from your colleague or friend.

As this answer is based on your own reflection, there is no outline answer at the end of the chapter.

You may now be thinking that there is an overlap between the role of coach and the practice assessment role you are experiencing in your practice learning, and you would be right. However, there are subtle differences, which we will look at in the next section.

Mentoring

Mentor was the name of a character in Greek mythology, the tutor of Odysseus' son Telemachus in Homer's *Odyssey*. The tutoring Mentor offered was not restricted to the giving of information; rather, he encouraged the exploration of subjects such as virtue, integrity, responsibility and character development. He was a trusted and wise counsellor. This historical meaning has remained in use over time and is still used today for someone who has acted as a role model or who has had a significant influence on a person's career or professional outlook on life. The term 'coach' is a more recent one and is used specifically to describe the growth in skills and knowledge toward a higher or improved level.

Confusingly, coaching can also be incorporated into a mentoring role. The term mentoring, today, can cover several roles, such as coach, adviser, guide, confidant/e, teacher, role model, counsellor, friend, consultant, critic and advocate. The NMC has identified standards for the practice *supervisors* and practice *assessors* (formerly called mentors, although we will use mentoring as a description of a form of management and leadership supporting and developing, and practice supervision and assessment when referring to the support and development of students) of nursing and midwifery students; these standards apply to already registered nurses who take on this role in addition to their day-to-day duties.

Activity 6.4   Evidence-based practice and research

Go to the website address in the useful websites section for the NMC *Standards to Support Learning and Assessing in Practice* and review the standards in section 2 for mentoring (in the future to be called practice supervision and assessment). Think about how you will undertake this role when you become a qualified nurse, and how you will plan to take a recognised practice supervision and assessment education programme.

This activity aims to help you understand more fully the role of practice supervising and assessing nursing students, but also encourages you to think about your own personal development plan as well as your engagement with the notion of lifelong learning.

You may want to discuss with your practice supervisor/assessor their experience of taking the practice supervision and assessing course and of being a practice supervisor and assessor to students. Reflect on what you can learn from your practice supervisor's experiences.

As a final part of this research activity, ask your practice supervisor if they had or have a practice supervisor now that they are qualified and, if so, what impact this has had on their working life.

As this answer is based on your own research and reflections, there is no outline answer at the end of the chapter.

Research summary: Multiprofessional views of mentorship

Bray and Nettleton (2007) researched the role of the mentor in nursing, midwifery and medicine using questionnaires and semi-structured telephone interviews with both mentors and mentees. They were interested in any differences in the professional perceptions of the role. They were also interested in the potential dilemma that mentors, who are perceived as wise guides, have to become assessors and make judgements on their mentees' abilities. This could be viewed as a conflict of interest. They found that for nurse mentors, the roles of teacher, supporter and role model were most important, with only 5 per cent indicating assessor as part of the role. By contrast, in midwifery the role of facilitator came higher than teacher and similarly few regarded assessor as part of the role. Within medicine, adviser and supporter were regarded as most important, with only 2 per cent regarding assessing as important.

When asked about any aspect of the role they found most difficult, both nurses and midwives reported difficulties in being objective toward their students when they had become 'supportive friends'. In medicine, less difficulty was reported with the assessor role. The biggest difficulty was finding time to commit to the role and all its aspects.

Bray and Nettleton found that across the professions there was a lack of clarity about the combination of the role of assessor with mentor. They admit that they had a small sample and have reservations about the **generalisability** of their findings. Yet, they make an interesting observation that, as we move toward further collaboration within multidisciplinary professional teams, a multiprofessional approach should be adopted toward defining the role and function of mentoring in healthcare professional education.

The confusion about the nature and purpose of mentoring remains a perennial problem within nursing. Nowell et al. (2017) identify that even in academic institutions there is a lack of clarity about what mentorship means and its general purpose in the development of mentees. Benner et al. (2009) describe both the novice and the advanced beginner nurse as requiring a mentor. They see a mentor as someone, perhaps an experienced nurse, whose role it is to assist with defining situations, setting priorities and integrating practical knowledge into working situations. Being in a relationship with a mentor aids nurses in their development from novice to expert practitioners (Benner, 1984). Certainly, within the trainee model in the UK, the NMC have decided to split the role of the practice supervisor and assessor.

Mentoring in other contexts

While we may be familiar with mentoring and practice supervision and assessment in healthcare settings, it is worth noting that mentoring takes place in other sectors and organisations outside of healthcare. We can learn from these relationships, as they provide a contrast to the practice supervisor and assessor experienced in healthcare, as well as ideas for opportunities for service development and relationships.

This could be to develop entrepreneurial or business skills (see Chapter 7), or alternatively to enhance working in community settings or with third-sector or voluntary services groups in the fields of mental health and learning disabilities. One example can be in business-to-business relationships, where a mentor from a large organisation may work with a small organisation to advise on development and growth. In business-to-social enterprise relationships, organisations such as the Prince's Trust have mentors to guide young business starters who have received grants from the Trust. Similar to this are training schemes supported by the government.

Providing mentoring to special needs or community projects has become an important part of community university engagement schemes, where more personal or individually tailored mentors are matched to individuals (Schuetze and Inman, 2010). Working the other way around, business people can work with education (e.g. head teachers, universities and students) to advise on business skills. There are also 'buddying' schemes between first- and third-year students, which are another version of mentoring.

Broadly speaking there are three main types of mentor:

1. The corporate mentor, who is a guide or counsellor in someone's career from orientation into the company to senior management.

2. The qualification mentor, who is required by a professional organisation – such as the NMC – to guide candidates toward achieving a qualification, including NVQs and QCFs.

3. The community mentor, who acts as a guide or counsellor to individuals who may be disadvantaged, experiencing social exclusion or in a distressing situation.

Throughout these discussions, there has been a tacit acknowledgement that everyone needs access to guidance or experienced advice at several points in their professional lives. Returning to the model of development associated with the seminal work of Benner (1984), it is clear that even experienced nurses return to the role of the novice when they move to new areas of work or take on new roles.

The notion of lifelong learning, mentioned earlier, is highly relevant in nursing, where care may not change but clinical treatments are constantly evolving. Consequently, we need to be prepared to update our practice and ensure our practice is meeting the needs of the client group with whom we work. Gaining experience in a given field is one way to add to our skills and knowledge. Seeking the guidance of a clinically experienced practitioner is another means of reflecting and learning from everyday practice. Often termed clinical supervision, it is the focus of the next section.

Clinical supervision

Over the years there have been as many definitions of clinical supervision as there are people writing about it. The definition by Snowdon et al. (2017, p786) is simple and straight to the point; they see clinical supervision as *the provision of guidance of clinical practice for qualified health professionals by a more experienced health professional.* Snowdon et al. (2017) identify how supervision is an important professional development activity, and that the importance of clinical supervision lies in the fact that it is directly associated with improvements in clinical care.

In practice, clinical supervision consists of a more junior nurse being matched with a more experienced nurse who is not a direct assessor or appraiser, thus providing a basis for a trusting relationship to develop. The aim is to build up a relationship so that the clinical supervisor can be contacted in times of need, rather than just meeting at set times. This model may be suitable for busy acute adult care environments but may not suit all situations, specialties and fields of practice.

Activity 6.5   Critical thinking

Consider when you have had one-to-one supervision and when you have had supervision as part of a group. Now make a list of the pros and cons of each approach. Which did you prefer and why?

Further guidance is given on this activity at the end of the chapter.

There are very specific and different statutory requirements for supervision of midwives, and the NMC has standards for the selection and activities of supervisors of midwives. In mental health settings, clinical supervision was introduced into pre-registration education in 1994, and in 1995 the UK Central Council for Nursing and Midwifery (forerunner of the NMC) declared clinical supervision should occur in all fields of nursing and midwifery. The literature suggests that the number of nurses receiving clinical supervision varies between regions and specialties. Similarly, the length of time and training for providing supervision is variable.

There do seem to have been technical advances made in the delivery of clinical supervision in community settings using telephone conferencing and similar techniques. The COVID-19 pandemic has seen much clinical supervision move online, a move that engenders both positive and negative responses from many health and social care professionals (Miller, 2020). However, most of the research literature concerns the educational provision of clinical supervision in pre-registration nursing courses (Tuomikoski et al., 2020).

Employer organisations, and their influence on implementing a culture supportive of clinical supervision, are seen as crucial themes in the literature. The factors influencing levels of engagement in organisations appear to be the culture, availability of time, supervisor numbers and local factors. The role of the organisation in creating a culture of learning will be discussed next.

The learning organisation

Learning organisations are seen by many as the way in which organisations will have to manage their structures for the twenty-first century (Middleton et al., 2021). Up until the mid-1980s it was quite possible to have a successful organisation without mentioning the word *learning*. As we move further into the twenty-first century, there is a world of global information and technologically driven organisations. Speed will be important to communicate changes and information management systems are increasingly important, as we see in practice with electronic patient records, etc. The importance of information, information management and information sharing means people in healthcare and health and social care organisations need to learn to do things differently and in a more timely manner – a process which has sped up exponentially during the COVID-19 pandemic. New information is constantly becoming available, requiring new ideas to be adopted and skills and knowledge to be continuously updated.

In healthcare we have seen the implementation over the last 20 years of developments such as telemedicine, microsurgery, stem cell research, patient-held records, shared patient management systems and many other technological and pharmacological advances. In addition, there are constant pressures to reduce costs and maximise efficiencies, which have led to a short-term focus on immediate results and constant efforts to rationalise the number of employees in organisations.

There is a conflict, therefore, between the organisation's need to manage the learning potential of its employees actively, and the pressures to change employment practices and professional roles. Not surprisingly, there is a culture of resistance to change if professional status and roles are eroded or services are seen to be reduced.

Case study: Changing the skill mix

The scene is a community healthcare setting. Two new roles have been introduced into the health visiting team to improve the skill mix. Joan, a nursery nurse, is employed to carry out focused parenting skills training over six weeks with families, providing weekly support to learn new skills. Joan is also available for advice at child health clinics. Usha is a staff nurse who used to work on a children's ward. She has a children's nursing qualification and experience, and is now employed to perform three-month developmental checks in the home. She is also available for pre-school checks to work with the school nurses. This frees up time for Liz, Jamil and Frances (the three health visitors in the team) to deal with complex family cases and public health initiatives. These kinds of cases have become much more prevalent in their caseloads and, while they would like to continue with providing a service to all mothers and their families, they realise that they need to focus their specialist expertise on more complicated cases where they can give extra time. Liz, Jamil and Frances are encouraged to undertake specialist,

(Continued)

(Continued)

post-qualifying courses in child protection and public health. Joan (the nursery nurse) and Usha (the staff nurse) are also given the opportunity to go on to further training: Joan to become a registered nurse and Usha to become a registered community health visitor and public health nurse. The team manager and the organisation (as part of its staff development strategy) are prepared to sponsor them for future training for career development. This also supports the organisation's strategy for succession planning and maintaining a learning culture.

This is an example of where new roles have been introduced into the team that are less costly than the health visitors to employ, which means efficiencies have been made. But Joan and Usha have the potential and ability to make a significant contribution to the work of the team as well as supporting the notion of a learning culture. At the same time, the experience and skills of the health visitors, Liz, Jamil and Frances, are maximised and not diminished by the inclusion of new roles into the team.

It is always worth your while looking into the staff development strategy of the organisation you will go to work for after you qualify, to see what opportunities there are for you to develop promotion opportunities or a career pathway.

The main features of a learning organisation are:

- an increased focus on learning and development to ensure organisational effectiveness and a sustainable future;
- encouraging as many people as possible to become coaches, practice supervisors and assessors or clinical supervisors, to ensure learning takes place in the workplace;
- establishing training programmes in coaching, practice supervision and assessment and clinical supervision;
- generating a culture that accepts the need to move from current standards of performance to higher levels, to ensure continuous improvements in performance;
- supporting individuals with managing their own learning to develop their skills, maximise potential and enable a satisfactory work–life balance (adapted from Parsloe and Leedham, 2009).

Activity 6.6   Critical thinking

Imagine you are working in a hospice and your manager has asked you to take on responsibility for managing all student placements. This role means you have to think about the learning needs of students from a variety of professional backgrounds, paying special consideration to what they might need to learn while on placement with you. How will you develop the culture of the team so that your hospice becomes a *learning environment?*

Hints

1. Would you first find out what kind of students attend the hospice and who the practice supervisors and assessors are?
2. Would you undertake an informal survey of their views on how to create a learning environment and one that considers, and that would benefit, multidisciplinary team working if more than one profession is represented?
3. Would you draw on any of your positive learning experiences as a student in other settings?
4. Would you look for any evidence in the literature of other initiatives to create learning environments or evidence to support your initiative?
5. Would you draw up your ideas into a proposal, citing the advantages and disadvantages of your ideas, and a plan of implementation for discussion in the team meeting?

As this answer is based on your own research and reflections, there is no outline answer at the end of the chapter.

The adoption of a learning culture in any workplace is, in essence, a reflection on the values of that workplace. Van Breda-Verduijn and Heijboer (2016, p123) identify a learning culture as *a collective, dynamic system of basic assumptions, values and norms which direct the learning of people within an organization.* These values translate into the way people are themselves valued, supported and developed in the workplace; as we saw in our case study: changing the skill mix. Workplaces which value people, and their development, are likely to be workplaces that attain good standards in patient care (remember what we said about the clinical care benefits of clinical supervision), as opposed to workplaces where staff are not valued, and therefore the work they do is valueless to them as well. One of the values underpinning nursing is the desire to provide the best care possible, often expressed as the value of *striving for excellence.* This is best achieved by a motivated workforce working in an environment that rapidly adopts improved ways of working and new practices, such as are found in a learning organisation. In this respect, creating a learning organisation as a nurse leader is a reflection of the core values of nursing.

Burnout and work–life balance

Throughout this chapter we have discussed ways that leaders and managers can support team members and colleagues. With increasingly complex workloads and demanding resource pressures we have to consider the effects this can have on the working life of the individual. In extreme cases, staff may experience degrees of burn-out. It is important to recognise the early signs of burnout before it takes hold, and also to look at ways of creating a work setting with a philosophy of encouraging and supporting a healthy work–life balance.

Burnout

Burnout is defined as a prolonged response to chronic emotional and interpersonal stressors on the job. It is famously defined by Maslach (2003) as presenting as three overwhelming dimensions of emotional exhaustion, depersonalisation (feeling disconnected from others) and sense of a lack of personal accomplishment (feeling incapable and incompetent). Unlike acute stress reactions, which develop in response to specific situations, burnout is a cumulative reaction to work stressors; that is, it tends to be chronic and its onset is slow and perhaps, in some cases, hard to detect. The emphasis is on the process of gradual psychological erosion and the social outcomes, rather than physical outcomes, of this chronic exposure. Burnout is therefore the result of prolonged exposure to chronic interpersonal stressors. Exhaustion, cynicism and a sense of inefficacy are the predictors. However, other workplace factors, such as working in care-giving environments where there is a sense of giving with little regard for self, as well as reduced resources, have been found to compound the likelihood of burnout (Heeb and Haberey-Knuessi, 2014).

Research summary: Burnout

In 2006, Edwards and colleagues surveyed community mental health nurses using the Maslach Burnout Inventory (MBI) and the Manchester Clinical Supervision Scale (MCSS) to identify whether effective clinical supervision could have a positive effect on burnout. Their findings indicated on the MBI that 36 per cent of staff had high levels of emotional exhaustion, 12 per cent had high levels of depersonalisation and 10 per cent had low levels of personal accomplishment. Those nurses who had completed six sessions of clinical supervision scored lower MBI scores and higher scores on the MCSS, which indicated effective supervision (Edwards et al., 2006).

In their cross-sectional study of the influence of COVID-19 on nursing burnout, Manzano García and Ayala Calvo (2021) identified how issues with perceived resources, workload and social support were aggravated by the perceived threat from the pandemic and explained the burnout experienced by nursing staff.

We don't really know yet what the long-term impact of the COVID-19 pandemic will be on nurse burnout, but it is likely that our understanding of the causes and effects of burnout, as well as the means for better managing it, will increase in the coming months and years as more research is undertaken in this area.

Work–life balance

Linked to the subject of burnout is the more recent concept of work–life balance. This is about people having a measure of control over when, where and how they work. It is achieved when an individual's right to a fulfilled life inside and outside paid work is accepted and respected as the norm, to the mutual benefit of the individual, organisation and society. Striking a balance between the needs of the individual employee, customer and organisation demands the following:

- For employees: Different individuals will have different expectations and needs at different times in their life.
- For customers: Organisations need to respond to the demands of their customers if they are to continue to be successful.
- For organisations: Organisations need to be able to manage costs, maintain profitability and ensure that teams work effectively together.

In 2019, an estimated 75 per cent of mothers were in employment, 1.8 million families were single-parent families, and about 17 per cent of the population were involved in caring for a relative. By 2070 there will be 7.5 million more people over the age of 65 than there are now. The UK is an increasingly service-based economy and there is little sign of this trend declining or reversing (HM Government, 2018). As a result of these demographic and economic changes, demands on workers to juggle home life, health and happiness are greater in the twenty-first century than ever before and will continue to grow.

The stresses and strains on a reduced workforce pool supporting an increasingly old and frail population will doubtless increase over the next 50 years, and so ways of managing the work–life balance of employees will become increasingly important. Strategies for managing stress and supporting and developing staff will become more important at individual, team and organisational levels.

Some of the strategies we are starting to see emerge in workplaces to help with work–life balance include increased working time flexibility both within the workplace and remotely (where this is possible), with many employers offering variations on shift times, shift patterns, annualised and family-friendly contracts. Simple ideas, such as ensuring staff take their annual leave in reasonable chunks throughout the year to avoid becoming over tired, encouraging social activities including staff from the workplace and duvet days, all help create an atmosphere in which staff want to work. Many workplaces have reward schemes for long, or otherwise distinguished, service as well as rewarding staff who stay with increased holiday allowances, access to certificated education and discretionary bonuses, etc.

Workplaces that invest in their people can expect to reap some rewards in terms of:

- improved staff morale;
- better productivity and care;

- reduced sickness absence;
- reduced staff turnover;
- improved recruitment.

On a personal level, as you progress your nursing career there are things you can do in and out of work to protect yourself from stresses and strains. Self-management is an important part of personal and professional development both as a nurse and a leader of people. Some of the things you should consider include:

- working for an employer who values their staff – you can see this in the way people talk about and review workplaces online;
- learning to say no when you cannot do a task which is being assigned to you;
- accessing supervision and support when they are offered;
- taking your breaks at work and away from work;
- undertaking some form of exercise;
- eating properly – both at work and away;
- getting into a routine with sleep;
- practising mindfulness, yoga or similar interventions.

It may not always be possible to introduce all of the ideas identified above to a workplace; however, working creatively with the philosophy of creating a work–life balance in the workplace will go some way to improving difficult working lives.

Chapter summary

In this chapter you have explored three different methods of staff support and development which can improve staff performance as well as improve work–life balance. Coaching can be used to improve staff performance and problem-solving abilities. It does not have to be undertaken by an expert in the field of practice. Mentoring has many different forms and can include coaching. Clinical supervision is usually undertaken by an expert in the field around a specific area of knowledge and might be delivered one-to-one or to a group.

It is essential for twenty-first-century organisations to create a learning culture if they are to keep abreast of innovations, support staff morale and encourage personal development options. In addition, the pressures of contemporary life need to be ameliorated by initiatives to bring about a balance between work and personal life. Leaders at all levels in the organisation have a part to play in creating these environments. Environments of care are influenced directly by the way in which leaders exercise their values, which need to remain central to everything they do.

Activities: Brief outline answers

Activity 6.5 Critical thinking (p120)

Clinical supervision	Advantages	Disadvantages
• Group supervision	• More people seen at one time, saving time • A variety of ideas can be offered from different perspectives • Helps with team building	• Takes more people away from the clinical area at one time • Requires an experienced/ trained facilitator • May not meet everyone's specific needs
• One-to-one	• More personal and focused • Deeper trusting relationship can be established • Can specifically match specialty advice	• Could become too intense • Personalities may not match • More resources required for time

Further reading

Benner, P (1984) *From Novice to Expert: Excellence and Power in Clinical Nursing Practice.* Menlo Park: Addison-Wesley.

One of the most influential pieces of work on the development of the nursing student.

Dolan, B and Overend, A (2018) *A Nurse's Survival Guide to Leadership and Management on the Ward* (3rd edition). London: Elsevier

A very practical view of ward level management.

Koy, V, Yunibhand, J, Angsuroch, Y and Fisher, M (2017) Relationship between nursing care quality, nurse staffing, nurse job satisfaction, nurse practice environment, and burnout: literature review. *International Journal of Research in Medical Sciences,* 3 (8): 1825–31.

An interesting review of the causes of burnout in nursing.

Kühne, F, Maas, J, Wiesenthal, S and Weck, F (2019) Empirical research in clinical supervision: a systematic review and suggestions for future studies. *BMC Psychology,* 7: 54. https://doi. org/10.1186/s40359-019-0327-7

A thoughtful and thorough review of clinical supervision research.

Westergaard, J (2017) *An Introduction to Helping Skills: Counselling, Coaching and Mentoring.* London: Sage.

A good primer on the approaches identified in this chapter.

Useful websites

www.cipd.co.uk/knowledge/fundamentals/people/development/coaching-mentoring-factsheet#7002

The CIPD's fact sheets on all things coaching and mentoring.

http://rapidbi.com/created/learningstyles.html#honeymumfordlearningstyleslsq

Learning styles review: several learning styles theories are displayed on this URL; however, the overview of Honey and Mumford's four learning styles – activist, reflector, theorist and pragmatist – will be particularly helpful for Activity 6.1.

www.nmc-uk.org/Educators/Standards-for-education/Standards-to-support-learning-and-assessment-in-practice

This link will take you to the NMC *Standards to Support Learning and Assessing in Practice*. See section 2.1 for the standards for mentorship – the old term for practice supervision and assessment.

www.princes-trust.org.uk

The Prince's Trust, which has mentors to guide young starters who have received grants from the Trust.

www.gov.uk/browse/working/finding-job

Similar to the above are training schemes supported by the government, as detailed on this site.

Chapter 7 Improving care and change management

NMC Standards of Proficiency for Registered Nurses

This chapter will address the following platforms and proficiencies:

Platform 1: Being an accountable professional

Registered nurses act in the best interests of people, putting them first and providing nursing care that is person-centred, safe and compassionate. They act professionally at all times and use their knowledge and experience to make evidence-based decisions about care. They communicate effectively, are role models for others, and are accountable for their actions. Registered nurses continually reflect on their practice and keep abreast of new and emerging developments in nursing, health and care.

At the point of registration, the registered nurse will be able to:

1.7 demonstrate an understanding of research methods, ethics and governance in order to critically analyse, safely use, share and apply research findings to promote and inform best nursing practice.

1.8 demonstrate the knowledge, skills and ability to think critically when applying evidence and drawing on experience to make evidence-informed decisions in all situations.

Platform 3: Assessing needs and planning care

Registered nurses prioritise the needs of people when assessing and reviewing their mental, physical, cognitive, behavioural, social and spiritual needs. They use information obtained during assessments to identify the priorities and requirements for person-centred and evidence-based nursing interventions and support. They work in partnership with people to develop person-centred care plans that take into account their circumstances, characteristics and preferences.

(Continued)

(Continued)

At the point of registration, the registered nurse will be able to:

3.11 undertake routine investigations, interpreting and sharing findings as appropriate.

3.12 interpret results from routine investigations, taking prompt action when required by implementing appropriate interventions, requesting additional investigations or escalating to others.

Platform 4: Providing and evaluating care

Registered nurses take the lead in providing evidence-based, compassionate and safe nursing interventions. They ensure that care they provide and delegate is person-centred and of a consistently high standard. They support people of all ages in a range of care settings. They work in partnership with people, families and carers to evaluate whether care is effective and the goals of care have been met in line with their wishes, preferences and desired outcomes.

At the point of registration, the registered nurse will be able to:

4.3 demonstrate the knowledge, communication and relationship management skills required to provide people, families and carers with accurate information that meets their needs before, during and after a range of interventions.

Platform 6: Improving safety and quality of care

Registered nurses make a key contribution to the continuous monitoring and quality improvement of care and treatment in order to enhance health outcomes and people's experience of nursing and related care. They assess risks to safety or experience and take appropriate action to manage those, putting the best interests, needs and preferences of people first.

At the point of registration, the registered nurse will be able to:

6.4 demonstrate an understanding of the principles of improvement methodologies, participate in all stages of audit activity and identify appropriate quality improvement strategies.

6.7 understand how the quality and effectiveness of nursing care can be evaluated in practice, and demonstrate how to use service delivery evaluation and audit findings to bring about continuous improvement.

6.9 work with people, their families, carers and colleagues to develop effective improvement strategies for quality and safety, sharing feedback and learning from positive outcomes and experiences, mistakes and adverse outcomes and experiences.

6.11 acknowledge the need to accept and manage uncertainty, and demonstrate an understanding of strategies that develop resilience in self and others.

Chapter aims

After reading this chapter you will be able to:

- describe different organisational structures;
- appreciate organisational requirements to maintain standards;
- compare change theories and their use in the change-management process;
- evaluate the appraisal tools available to improve work performance;
- appreciate a new approach to changing practice through entrepreneurial skills.

Introduction

This chapter will help you understand how organisations are structured and operate to maintain and improve standards. It considers the structure and practice of organisational clinical governance and explores how you can contribute to change management. Included in this chapter is a discussion of methods used to improve standards of working through performance appraisal, supervision and 360-degree reviews. The final section looks at how entrepreneurial nurses can use a business-minded approach to improving patient care.

Understanding your organisation

Once qualified, you will be busy adapting to your new responsibilities and accountabilities and getting to grips with a new working environment. You will have little time to think about the 'powers that be' or the 'upper echelons' of the organisational structure in which you work. But as this structure has an impact on your daily working life it is worth spending a few minutes figuring out who controls what.

Organisational structures influence the way they operate and perform. The structure, which will vary according to the mission and culture of the organisation, provides a framework for distributing responsibilities for the different activities the organisation undertakes between the different services, departments and individuals. Factors influencing the shape of this structure include organisational size, main purpose and skills of the workforce. The historical origins of a hospital (e.g. as a Victorian workhouse) or location (e.g. in an industrial area, close to a medieval leper colony or monastery), although distant from the modern demands of current NHS or private-sector healthcare, may nevertheless influence the organisation's culture.

Activity 7.1   Evidence-based practice and research

1. Ask your practice supervisor if they know the origins of the organisation where you are currently on placement. Consider whether this has had any impact on the functions of the organisation today.
2. Go to the web page of the organisation and look for the welcome page. See if there is a strapline which outlines the main priorities of the organisation. There may be a statement which says 'Our main objective is to …' or 'Our mission is to …'; often the best place to look for this is within the 'about us' section. Finding these key messages helps you understand what the priorities are. Each organisation will produce an annual report; whether they have a web page or not, this is a good place to look for the vision and mission of the organisation, as well as identifying its structure and plans for the future. Seek this out to see what the main priorities for the organisation are.

As this answer is based on your own research and reflections, there is no specimen answer at the end of the chapter.

An important factor in any organisational structure, whether historically derived, a private healthcare company or small-scale organisation (such as a charitable foundation supporting a hospice), is the **span of control**. Used to describe the number of employees each organisation manager or head of department is responsible for, this can also be expressed in financial terms, such as the budget or annual financial turnover of a department. The span of control will determine issues such as the structure, number of departments and managers in an organisation. There will usually be a chief executive (although occasionally organisations have more than one), managing director or hospital director or similar post, and a governing board with a number of board members, some of whom will be external to the organisation to provide expert advice or represent other organisations. In the NHS, for example, these would be patient organisation and local authority representatives from the council or regional government offices.

Activity 7.2   Evidence-based practice and research

Find out the structure in the organisation you have a placement in or hope to work in when you qualify. Try to get hold of a copy of the structure or ask your mentor to sketch one out.

Identify who sits on the board of the organisation, as this is the main decision-making body with the power to agree or prevent service developments; also usually found within the 'about us' section of the website.

Find out if there is a nurse member of the board who represents your professional interests.

As this answer is based on your own research and reflections, there is no specimen answer at the end of the chapter.

Organisation structure

The Learn Management website (**www.learnmanagement2.com**) describes five main organisational structures: tall, flat, hierarchical, matrix and centralised/decentralised. On this website you will find descriptions of each type of structure, along with some of its advantages and disadvantages. In brief, a *tall* structure is one that has many levels of management, with each line manager having a small number of people reporting directly to him or her, so that the people on the lower levels may have no contact at all with those higher up. This can have implications for accountability and communication, but it does provide employees with a clear management structure with ample opportunities for promotion.

By contrast, a *flat* structure has fewer management layers, but each manager has quite a large number of people (all at more or less the same level) reporting to them. This can encourage team spirit and a sense of collective belonging, but it can be difficult to manage if the organisation is large. A *hierarchical* organisation has much in common with a tall organisation, but there are likely to be more people reporting directly to managers on each different level, particularly at the lower levels (thus giving them a pyramid shape). The most important decisions tend to be taken by the most senior people.

The *matrix* structure could not be more different. In an organisation with this type of structure, the important unit is the team. Each team will be led by a project manager or team leader and will be responsible for a specific project or aspect of the organisation's work. In some organisations, the team will only exist for the duration of the work required by the project (e.g. a team of healthcare professionals and managers setting up a new clinic). In others, the team becomes an established department within a whole organisation structure (e.g. the people who will run the clinic). In many cases, the matrix organisation would consist of a mixture of permanent teams and project-specific teams.

Tall structures can be contrasted with flat structures, and hierarchical organisations with matrix-based organisations. Another important contrast is between centralised and decentralised structures. In a *centralised* organisation, a small group of senior managers (or a 'head office', which will be in a specific location) retains the major responsibilities and powers. In a *decentralised* organisation, these powers are devolved down to various lower-level managers, perhaps spread over a wide geographical area. Foundation trusts are excellent examples of the decentralised structure. Each trust is a management unit in itself, but, although the executive board is relatively autonomous on a day-to-day basis, they will be ultimately answerable to NHS England and the Department of Health and Social Care – either directly or through an agency such as the Care Quality Commission.

Some organisations may find a combination of centralisation and decentralisation to be most effective. For example, functions such as accounting or warehousing may be centralised to save costs. The Department of Health and Social Care uses a mixture of centralisation and decentralisation, with central policy decisions being made to influence local health services. At the same time, local NHS Trusts have functions and responsibilities to respond to local population health needs and to manage their organisations according to the workforce they require to deliver those services. One further example of this is the UK Health Security Agency, which is an executive agency of the Department of Health and Social Care and has a UK-wide remit for public health and infectious disease protection, but the responsibility for public health lies with local authorities, which are autonomous in this respect and usually have their own director of public health.

Nurses at board level

An influential government report in the early 1980s observed that, *If Florence Nightingale were carrying her lamp through the corridors of the NHS today, she would almost certainly be searching for the people in charge* (Griffiths, 1983). In the wake of this, the Royal College of Nursing launched a campaign with the slogan 'Nursing should be managed by nurses' and, indeed, the first nurse general managers were appointed shortly afterwards (*Nursing Standard*, 1985). Nurse managers should be well placed to improve the business of caring, by helping boards not only to understand the quality of care patients receive on the wards, but also to make positive decisions that improve care.

During the 1990s and early this millennium, the management of NHS organisations had started to focus on financial measures (e.g. cost management and budgets) and performance targets (e.g. waiting times and operations done) rather than on the quality of clinical care. However, the Darzi report (Darzi, 2008) has reversed this trend, describing the improvement in quality of care as *the basis of everything we do in the NHS*. The business of caring was brought to the forefront in the review and considered just as important as financial management. Although, as in any complex organisation, sometimes the message gets lost in translation, with Francis (2013) identifying that one of the key issues with the culture within the Mid Staffs NHS Trust was its continued focus on financial rather than care-driven targets.

Collectively, Darzi and Francis produce a raft of different issues for managers and leaders, especially in senior roles, where the emphasis has shifted from cost efficiency (i.e. money management) to effectiveness (i.e. good-quality care) to what is now more common in that they need to think of both. That is, the emphasis in modern healthcare management is on achieving both effectiveness and efficiency, the best care for the best price.

Nurses are now represented at board level in almost all healthcare facilities. The post of nurse executive (or nursing director) was established alongside the first wave of NHS Trusts in 1991. In 2007, the Burdett Trust commissioned the King's Fund to develop an intensive programme of work to support executive nurses and NHS boards in raising the quality of clinical care and giving a central place to patients and how they experience healthcare.

This work has resulted in two reports:

1. *From Ward to Board* (Machell et al., 2009) sets out the key questions and findings from the first phase of the programme and identifies good practice that can be easily replicated. Key areas to be built on are identified, along with the key skills and qualities nurse executives need to fulfil their role effectively.

2. *Putting Quality First in the Boardroom: Improving the Business of Caring* (Machell et al., 2010) is based on observations of how nurse executives and their boards work together. This report builds on themes that emerged from the previous one, and addresses long-standing concerns about the way in which financial and administrative performance indicators have taken precedence over issues relating to the quality of clinical care.

Commitment to the patient experience and the role of the NHS in the wider community is further recognised in the 2014 *Five Year Forward View* plan and in the 2019 *NHS Long Term Plan*, both published by NHS England, which reiterated this position, stating that patients and communities need to be at the heart of care. Other indicators of the NHS's commitment to improving the patient experience include the widespread use of satisfaction survey tools such as the 'Friends and Family Test' (NHS England, 2013).

Activity 7.3   Research and finding out

Go online and find a copy of the 'Friends and Family Test'. Consider how you might respond to the questions contained within it with regard to your last experience as a healthcare user, as well as how people might respond to it in the area you are currently working, or last worked.

As this answer is based on your own research and reflections, there is no specimen answer at the end of the chapter.

Governance

This section examines the regulatory bodies responsible for ensuring quality and good **governance** in health and social care organisations. The White Paper *Equity and Excellence: Liberating the NHS* (Department of Health, 2010) proposed changes to the governance, regulation and accountability arrangements of the NHS in England. The Care Quality Commission (CQC) is a regulatory body with responsibility for monitoring the quality of health and social care provision in England. It was created in 2009 through a merger of the Healthcare Commission, the Mental Health Commission and the Care Service Inspection Service. Scotland, Northern Ireland and Wales have separate governance arrangements.

Activity 7.4   Research and finding out

If you are in placement in any health or social care organisation in England there will have been a CQC inspection within recent years. This activity will help you find the most recent report. Go to the website: **www.cqc.org.uk**.

In the 'Search whole website' box put a place name or postcode and select a service you wish to find out about. Read the most recent report, paying special attention to the elements of quality as identified by the inspectorate, as well as the type of evidence to support the conclusions they have come to about the service. It is also useful to look back over old reports, as this gives you an idea if the service is one in which the quality of care is thought to be improving, staying the same or declining.

As this answer is based on your own research, there is no specimen answer at the end of the chapter.

Case study: Investigating quality of care

Cygnet Yew Trees was a small hospital providing care for women who had learning disabilities. In April of 2019, the CQC found, during a comprehensive inspection, that the hospital was not fulfilling its obligations relating to regulation 12 (safe care and treatment) of the Health and Social Care Act 2008 (Regulated Activities) Regulations 2014 (CQC, 2020).

In the November of the same year, they returned to undertake a focused inspection having received information of concern. They identified that the hospital was still in breach of regulation 12 and issued a requirement notice which obliged the managers to provide a report to the CQC about how they were going to address the concerns identified in the inspection. The service was placed in special measures in December 2019 – this means the facility is under scrutiny from the CQC and must follow a clearly identified plan for improvement.

In January of the following year, the CQC undertook another comprehensive inspection and identified breaches of The Health and Social Care Act 2008 (Regulated Activities) Regulations 2014 for regulation 12 (safe care and treatment), 16 (receiving and acting on complaints) and 17 (good governance). At this point they imposed conditions on the hospital's registration.

In September 2020, during a focused inspection, they found serious concerns relating to breaches of The Health and Social Care Act 2008 (Regulated Activities) Regulations 2014 for regulation 12 (safe care and treatment), 13 (safeguarding service users from abuse and improper treatment), 17 (good governance) and 18 (staffing). In October, the CQC effectively closed Cygnet Yew Trees as a provider.

In their reports the CQC identified how:

- staff did not protect service users from abuse;
- staff did not report abuses;
- staff failed to record incidents;
- management failed to manage the health and safety of service users;
- managers did not act on audit findings;
- managers did not recruit safely and failed to provide robust supervision of staff;
- there was a culture of abuse in the hospital.

Because the management failed to address the issues with the culture of the hospital and failed to keep people safe, the culture of the hospital deteriorated to such an extent that it was deemed unsafe for patients.

This real-life case illustrates the power of the CQC and its ability to act swiftly and responsively if concerns are raised about a regulated service.

Concept summary: Governance

The term governance is widely used throughout all aspects of life. In health and social care, the term **clinical governance** is heard almost every day. At its simplest, clinical governance promotes good practice. There are, however, as many definitions of what clinical governance is as there are people writing about it.

The term clinical governance initially emerged in the White Paper 'The New NHS: Modern and Dependable' (Department of Health, 1997) and came into effect in 1998 being, as it was, central to ongoing NHS reform. Later its principles were more widely adopted for use in the healthcare sector (see the Health and Social Care Act, 2008).

Brennan and Flynn (2013) suggest clinical governance is a way of promoting integrated quality improvement across administrative and clinical functions within a framework providing the basis for clinical accountability and clinical professional performance. Therefore, all activity that challenges, promotes and records professional practice (including performance, continuing professional development and regulatory activity), fall within the remit of clinical governance.

Improving standards

Improving the quality of clinical care occurs at many levels, organisationally, within services, within teams and individually. NHS Improvement (formed in 2016) exists specifically to support foundation trusts and NHS trusts *to give patients consistently safe, high quality, compassionate care within local health systems that are financially sustainable* (NHS

Improvement, 2016, p2). This is achieved through providing strategic leadership and practical help to the sector, supporting and *holding providers to account* to achieve a single definition of success (NHS Improvement, 2016, p2). Healthcare Improvement Scotland fulfils a similar role.

Activity 7.5   Evidence-based practice and research

Go online and find the King's Fund website. The King's Fund is an independent charity that works toward improving health and care provision in England. Find its publications page and look out the 2016 report 'Improving Quality in the English NHS'. Consider what it says are its key findings about what is needed to improve the quality of care provided by the NHS in England.

As this answer is based on your own research, there is no specimen answer at the end of the chapter.

In Chapter 6, we discussed how staff development could enable individuals to develop their skills further. Performance review (often also called appraisal) is one method that managers use to regulate how well individuals carry out their responsibilities. The Chartered Institute of Personnel and Development (CIPD, 2020) claims it is important to distinguish between performance management and performance review. Performance management is undertaken through supervision, and achievements are observed against a specific set of objectives or goals, whereas performance review is a dialogue between manager and subordinate to discuss an individual's performance, past and future development and the support required from the organisation and manager to achieve optimum performance. Armstrong-Stassen et al. (2015) suggest, when seen to be undertaken fairly, the process of performance appraisal can also be a motivator for staff retention. In this sense, performance appraisal is a tool to be used in performance management.

The CIPD (2020) recommends that performance reviews contain the following elements.

1. Measurement – assessing the performance against agreed targets and objectives which are kept to a minimum and which are SMART (Specific, Measurable, Achievable (yet stretching), Relevant and Time-bound).

2. Feedback – providing information to individuals on their performance and progress as part of a two-way process.

3. Strengths based – emphasising what has been done well and making only constructive criticism about what might be improved using their reflections on what works well.

Appraisal tools

There are several tools that can be used for performance appraisal. The simplest is a trait-rating scale, where individuals are rated using a numerical score against a set of standards, including their job description, knowledge, behaviours and personal traits – such as attitude to work. This method invites a subjective decision, which is open to potential bias, and, if a point scale is used, a tendency to score to the mid-line, making the process meaningless.

Self-assessment methods involve individuals submitting a portfolio of achievements and productivity. While introspection and self-awareness can result in growth and achievement, feedback on achievements is essential for a positive result.

Management by objectives is a technique seldom used in healthcare. It incorporates a process that negotiates both the organisation's objectives and the individual's assessments. It is a very specific form of appraisal, with individuals measured against the objectives on a regular basis. In public healthcare organisations, the appraisal is usually an annual event, whereas management by objectives is often quarterly and therefore far more intensive and oriented toward action by observable results.

Peer review is, as the name suggests, a process whereby professional colleagues monitor and assess each other's performance. It is used widely in medicine and education, and less widely in wider healthcare. The NMC uses this approach to review nursing and midwifery education. Peer review events take place on an annual basis with a group of colleagues from other, similar organisations or professional groups conducting a review of systems and processes set against publicly available criteria. The process requires data to be collected from a variety of sources, such as charts, patient care plans, information systems, other professionals and patients.

An adaptation of the peer review process is 360-degree feedback. This is an assessment of performance that provides information from a variety of sources and often includes a group of colleagues who work with an individual (CIPD, 2020). Usually, eight to ten people complete questionnaires that can also include a self-assessment, and which are submitted anonymously to an independent observer to collate the responses into a report for the individual. The report should demonstrate a synthesis of information about performance in a role. In healthcare, this could include patients as well as co-workers to provide all-round information, which is where the name originates. This allows the individuals being assessed to understand how other people view them (as in the Johari window, discussed in Chapter 1), and can enable the developing leader to work on areas of their behaviour of which they might otherwise not be aware.

We have previously discussed clinical supervision and coaching (Chapter 6) as a means of supporting individuals to develop new skills. These are also tools that a manager can utilise to improve work performance and standards.

It is worth at this stage reflecting on the nature and purpose of the various means by which people might be appraised and considering their respective strengths and weaknesses. These are set out in Table 7.1.

	Advantages	Disadvantages
Clinical supervision	Personal and focused	Could become too intense
	Deeper trusting relationship can be established	Personalities may not match
		More resources required for time
	Can specifically match specialty area to improve performance	
Coaching	Personalised	Takes time
	Identifies specific goals	Needs in-depth coaching training to be effective
	Enhances personal motivation	
Trait-rating scales	Uses a set standard that is transparent	Can lead to subjective assessments
		Central tendency in scores
	Incorporates personal behaviours such as attitudes	'Halo' or 'horns' effects from rater
Self-appraisal	Collects examples of impact on standards and is achievement-oriented	Gives little scope for feedback – positive or negative
	Enables personal growth and awareness	May have focused on goals that do not correspond to organisational targets for improvement
Management by objectives	Determines individual progress, incorporating both employee and organisation's goals	Authoritarian and directive managers find this approach difficult due to the negotiated nature of the goal setting
	Promotes individual growth and excellence	Some employees may set easily achievable goals
Peer review	Has the potential to increase accuracy of performance appraisal, as collects data from wider range of sources	Requires high levels of trust to share data
		More time consuming than one-to-one appraisals
	Can enhance team working and improve understanding between different teams, especially interdisciplinary teams	Takes time to orient staff to the process, requires training and has high administration costs
	Provides increased opportunities for professional learning and sharing of good practice	Shifts authority away from manager, which can be threatening to the manager, who may feel exposed
360-degree appraisal	Feedback from a variety of sources	Requires questionnaires to be designed and administered, data collected anonymously and collated into a report, which is costly and time consuming
	Provides a broader perspective on an individual's performance	
		Could be threatening to have such a wide selection of subjective opinions about an individual's performance

Table 7.1 Comparison of appraisal methods

> ## Activity 7.6   Reflection and critical thinking
>
> You may not have had an appraisal in the sense discussed here, but you will have been assessed by your practice supervisor and/or practice assessor. They will, for instance, look at your accomplishment of some of the skills required of the 'future nurse' (NMC, 2018a) and judge your performance against the description of the procedures and skills it describes. How do you feel about being appraised in this way? What are the best experiences of appraisal you have had, and what are the worst? Consider why the process was good or bad and how you might manage the process of giving feedback when you are the person doing the assessing.
>
> *Further guidance is given on this activity at the end of the chapter.*

Rewards

Performance appraisal can also be used as a means of assessing an individual's ability to be promoted or moved to another pay band. The now simplified Knowledge and Skills Framework, defined in the Agenda for Change (AfC) pay agreement (**www.nhsemployers.org/SimplifiedKSF**), paved the way for a Gateway Policy to be formulated by NHS Trusts to ensure that staff covered by the AfC would obtain a transparent opportunity to move to a higher pay band. Under the AfC, progression from one pay point to another is assessed each year against the skills identified in the Knowledge and Skills Framework bands. At defined points, known as Gateways, management decisions will be made about progression to higher levels of pay and responsibility. There are two Gateways in each of the nine pay bands: Foundation, which takes place no later than 12 months after an individual is appointed to a pay band, and Second Gateway, which is set at a fixed point toward the top of a pay band.

Planning change

Change, or service improvement, is a constant feature of health and social care. Changes are sometimes driven by policies to restructure organisations, by improvements in medical science such as the development of stem cell research, or advances in society's attitudes to rights, such as with the Human Rights Act (1998) and changes in legislation such as the Mental Capacity Act (2005). In the day-to-day running of a ward or unit, the types of change that take place can be personal (such as when staff change) or organisational (such as changes in shift patterns) or the way in which internal services are delivered (e.g. bed management, portering services, catering services or discharge-planning methods).

There are many forces driving change in healthcare that are not just related to the UK. Rising costs of medical treatments, shortages of skilled workforces, increasing technology, availability of information and a growing elderly population have led, in some cases, to extreme destabilisation and a constant need to upgrade structures, promote better quality and manage workforce constraints. Whatever the changes to the work environment, there are those who embrace the changes and those who find it very difficult to adapt. As a result of the COVID-19 pandemic, many of the health and social care practices in the UK have had to change both quickly and dramatically, with an increased emphasis on infection control and the use of protective masks. Nurses in the future will need to be even more adaptable than they have been in the past to keep up with changes and adapt to the new challenges of a world in which coronaviruses are a daily reality.

Activity 7.7   Reflection

What is your personal perspective on change? Below is a short rating scale for you to self-assess your attitude to change. Place a mark in the score that most fits your perspective: 1 = low agreement; 5 = high agreement.

	1	2	3	4	5
1. I always embrace change					
2. I look for opportunities to change things					
3. I accept change reluctantly					
4. I avoid change at all costs					
5. My response to change is the same as that of my friends and family					
6. Have you always responded to change in this way, or have you changed in your lifetime?					
7. What events have altered your views and responses to change?					

As this answer is based on your own experience and reflections, there is no specimen answer at the end of the chapter.

Initiating and co-ordinating change requires well-developed leadership and management skills. It requires vision and expert planning skills because neither skill alone is sufficient.

Many of the best ideas for changing practice fail because of inadequate preparation and planning. Poor preparation results in problems during implementation, frustrated staff and lack of successful outcome. Others fail at the first hurdle or later in the process because the team, the people having to implement and live with the change, do not understand the vision – there is a lack of clarity about what the change is meant to achieve.

Change theory

Most of the contemporary research into change management originates from the work of social psychologist Kurt Lewin in the mid-twentieth century. There are other theories; however, we will concentrate on Lewin's theory in this book and will compare it briefly with newer developments in complexity theory and chaos theory. If you are interested in other theories, please go to the useful websites at the end of this chapter for further information.

Lewin (1951) identified three stages through which change must proceed before any planned change will become embedded in an organisation or system of working. The stages are unfreezing, movement and refreezing.

Unfreezing is when the change agent proposes a convincing plan for change to the team or management. It is also when team members who are not keen on the change can be helped to draw out their anxieties or concerns about the change. At this stage people become either discontented about the proposal or increasingly aware of the need to change. The skilful leader will be able to work with these conflicting views to build up trust in the change proposal's worth and the value of putting effort into the proposed change. Nelson-Brantley and Ford (2017) identify how enabling individual and team leadership, providing support and developing and maintaining working relationships are all important in the change-management process. They further identify how change is driven by factors internal and external to the organisation, and that organisational culture is an important aspect of readiness for change.

During unfreezing, leaders need to take account of the balance between change and stability. Too much change leads to instability, which results in feelings of lack of control, insecurity and anxiety. A good leader will assess the relative merits of the forces for and against change, such as extent of the proposed change, nature and depth of motivation of **stakeholders** and the environment in which the change will occur; this last could be physical (e.g. buildings) or political (e.g. local or national policy). Burnes (2017) identifies that people often oppose change, and while this is sometimes legitimate in that the change is perhaps ill advised, one of the roles of the change manager is to shift the emphasis from imposition of, to participation in, change. In many instances, this is about how the change agent makes the goals of the change obvious, so that people who are resisting understand what is trying to be achieved and buy into the process.

In the second stage there is *movement* toward accepting the change, and a plan of action and implementation is instigated. Change takes time as people adjust to the idea, come to understand the benefits of the change and eventually become adopters of the change. This cannot be achieved unless the change agent has been successful in persuading people of the need for the change in the unfreezing stage.

The final stage, according to Lewin (1951), is *refreezing*. Change needs time before it is accepted as part of the system. This means that, after the change is implemented, support will still be needed to embed the change. The leader's role is to help the continued integration of the change into practice to ensure refreezing – that is, the change becoming part of normal practice; if this does not occur, people will revert to doing what they did before.

A good way of understanding Lewin's theory is to think of how you might create a spherical ice block from a cube shaped one. There are two main approaches to achieving this. The first is to chip away and try to achieve the change in shape. This is time consuming, takes effort and the outcome is not guaranteed. The second approach is to melt the ice cube, pour the resulting water into a new mould and refreeze it. This approach is simple and guarantees that the desired result is achieved.

One method to ensure the effects of change are perceived as beneficial is to measure the outcomes of change or make improvements to the change as a result of feedback from outcome measures. Thus, a plan to evaluate the change should be incorporated in the overall change-management plan.

Steps of change

Stage 1: Unfreezing

1. Gather data and information about the planned change.

2. Accurately and objectively describe the issues that are causing the problem or reason for change. Use evidence and hard facts, not supposition or 'finger in the air' tactics.

3. Decide whether change is really needed and identify the reasons for change. This could be a pilot for your ideas by testing on your team or one or two close colleagues.

4. Make others aware of the need for change. This also involves highlighting discontent with the current system, i.e. what is wrong or not productive. Progress to the next stage should not happen until sufficient discontent is expressed about the current system.

Stage 2: Movement

1. Develop a change-management plan – this could take the form of a project plan (use a **Gantt chart** if it will help you visualise what you want to achieve – see Further reading at the end of the chapter).

2. Set goals and objectives.

3. Identify areas of support and resistance.

4. Include everyone who will be affected by the change in its planning; however, you may want to have a small project group or reference group to help manage the project with you.

5. Set target dates and timelines.

6. Develop appropriate strategies.

7. Implement the change.

8. Be available to support others and offer encouragement through the change process.

9. Use strategies for overcoming resistance to change.

10. Evaluate the change.

11. Modify the change if necessary.

Stage 3: Refreezing

Support others so that the change is sustainable and remains in place to achieve improved outcomes (adapted from Marquis and Huston (2020), p195).

Another change-management, or process-improvement model, which is widely used in health and social care settings, is the PDSA model or cycle, where the letters stand for:

- **P**lan
- **D**o
- **S**tudy
- **A**ct

This simple cycle shares some common features with the nursing process of assess, plan, implement and evaluate, in that it is in a continuous improvement cycle. Like Lewin's model of change management, the PDSA cycle involved stages of planning, doing and, once the change is working, refreezing or acting.

Case study: Change management

Ross and Meier (2021) identify how they used the PDSA cycle in their change project to help adults cope with the effects of social isolation during the COVID-19 pandemic, using various telehealth interventions. Their project required four cycles of PDSA and involved a survey stage to identify the issues, an implementation stage utilising telehealth and written information, and a cycle involving telehealth and listening.

The driving force for the change was the need to support people who had a need for nursing input into their care, but to do it remotely to reduce their risks of contracting COVID-19. What they found by following a multistage process for their change project was that people needed their health education and support delivered in different ways using remote tele-health methods. This demonstrates the value of the cyclical process of change management in that this person-centred approach was able to simultaneously deliver and evaluate the telehealth approaches used in a way which might not have been possible using a single-phase change-management model.

Activity 7.8   Decision-making

Identify a change you would like to make in your personal life. List the driving forces that you think are your reasons for wanting to change. Then list the restraining forces that you think will inhibit you making the change. Work out a plan, utilising all of the steps of change in the box above, to achieve the change.

Hint

Remember the driving forces will need to exceed your reluctance to change and you will need to feel sufficient discontent with how things currently are for the change process to tip from unsuccessful to successful. You will also need to plan time for the change to be embedded into your everyday life. This means it will take longer than you originally planned; especially if you were hoping for quick results.

As this answer is based on your own decision-making, there is no specimen answer at the end of the chapter.

Complexity theory and chaos theory

Lewin's change theory is a linear approach to change, with an optimistic view that change, once implemented, will be refrozen and equilibrium re-established. In this current world, where science is moving the frontiers of knowledge forward at an increasing pace and organisations respond to change more rapidly, the linear approach may not always work. This is particularly evident in world healthcare in 2021, where approaches to the management of the COVID-19 pandemic have had to change rapidly, to keep pace with the increases in understanding about how the virus works, moves between people and mutates. Consequently, non-linear change theories, such as complexity theory and chaos theory, now influence contemporary thinking about change.

Complexity theory maintains that we inhabit a complex world where individuals are multifaceted, and situations are forever dynamic and changing. The theory originates from physics, where the natural order of science is challenged by systems that are constantly adapting because of the interaction between parts and feedback loops that change things and do not maintain the status quo. An example of this is that an individual may have behaved in a certain way in the past, but that person's future behaviour may not be predictably the same.

Olson and Eoyang (2001) developed a theory of complex adaptive systems, which maintains that we should not focus on the large changes taking place but on the effects of change at a micro level between individuals. It is at the individual level where relationships, and simple expressions of rules, are responsible for change. When applying this theory to changes in healthcare it suggests we should concentrate on the individuals who work in the organisations and understand these relationships before attempting to unfreeze, as in Lewin's theory. They also suggest that continual monitoring and adaptation are needed for refreezing to be achieved.

Research summary: Complexity theory and organisations

Storkholm et al. (2019) undertook a study, informed by complexity theory, which considered the quality improvement changes made in an obstetric and gynaecology service. They undertook reviews of documents and interviewed 30 staff, including 12 regular staff and 12 departmental managers, as well as undertaking in excess of 250 hours of observation. The interviews collected data about the context for the changes, the processes which the changes followed and the content of the changes themselves. They used the data collected to analyse the process of the changes, employing a complexity analysis framework.

The researchers discovered that the process of change was actually a multiplicity of changes. They found that 53 individually identifiable changes had been made as part of the change process. They saw how the process was adaptive and changed according to what they discovered as the quality initiative progressed. Storkholm et al. (2019) illustrated how an iterative (i.e. a 'test it and see') approach to the changes was undertaken in following a 'professional path' with management and staff implementing and analysing the impact of each step using a process-mapping approach. They showed how allowing the process to be 'complicated' enabled the team to identify the developmental opportunities and find solutions to issues as the project progressed.

Chaos theory was first described in 1963 by Edward Lorenz, a meteorologist working on the problem of weather predictability. It is related to complexity theory in that it refers to the unpredictable and adaptive factors that affect events. Lorenz discovered that a minor change in a part of an experiment could change the whole outcome. A practical example is where a slight rise in the temperature of the ocean in one place in the world may have an effect on the airflow that will eventually lead to a change in temperature in another part of the world.

Chaos theory helps us understand why a small change in a situation can alter how a system functions. Chaos theory also suggests that it is impossible to know what this change may be, because there are so many different variables that can affect a situation. For example, even if you know everything about an infectious disease – how it is transmitted, how to slow transmission and who is worst affected by it – you still cannot accurately predict how it will act in the real world, because how people will behave is itself not predictable. That said, as understanding of the disease grows, some elements of its behaviour will become easier to predict.

The application of complexity theory to change management in organisations provides a means of understanding why change does not always go to plan because of unpredictable multifactorial influences and, second, that understanding small effects, as chaos theory suggests, can have a big effect in a change-management plan. For example, individuals who do not trust the change plan or do not think it can work could jeopardise it. However, if they are brought into the change process and their ideas given a hearing, they may not feel the need to jeopardise the plan. A major lesson for managers is that they cannot completely control a change plan because there will always be some elements that cannot be predicted in advance that will affect it. Managers need to learn how to manage the anxiety that accompanies change as well as flexibility and the ability to think on their feet so that they can manage the unexpected. In Chapter 9 we talk some more about the impact of change on individuals and their self-esteem.

There is, of course, a further complication within healthcare and nursing: people. As well as staff, of which there are many professions and grades operating within any one team, patients are all unique. The uniqueness of individuals and increasing awareness of healthcare rights and responsibilities can mean that different people will ask, and deliver, different things even in the same circumstances. People are complex, and their unpredictable responses to challenges and change can provoke chaos even within the best managed system.

Living in a constantly changing world where there is rapid technological, social, cultural and political change, we have to be prepared to adapt, be willing to learn and test our assumptions. Things that worked in the past may not work in the future and nurses have always been able to find new ways of managing problems and being creative. That is why, in the next section, we will explore how nurses can use this creativity to improve patient care.

Tools for change: entrepreneurship

In the UK, there has been limited uptake of independent practitioners of nursing and midwifery; however, the skills of entrepreneurship are now being debated as a potential, valuable contribution to innovative healthcare initiatives. From an extensive literature review, da Silva Copelli et al. (2019) found three levels at which nurses act as entrepreneurs and identify the three different types of nursing entrepreneur.

1. Social entrepreneur: an individual who assumes the total responsibility and risk for discovering or creating unique opportunities to use personal talents, skills and energy, and who employs a strategic planning process to transfer that opportunity into a marketable service or product.
2. Nurse entrepreneur: a proprietor of a business that offers nursing services of a direct care, educational, research, administrative or consultative nature. The self-employed nurse provides a service directly to the client and is entirely autonomous.

3. Nurse intrapreneur: nurses who have a job of work for which they are paid, but who seek out new ways of working and innovate ideas within the organisation.

It is this last role that we will be exploring in this chapter. Within these definitions it is clear that the only difference between an intrapreneur and entrepreneur is the setting in which the skills of entrepreneurship are used.

The NMC (2018a) *Future Nurse: Standards of Proficiency for Registered Nurses* Platform 6 'Improving safety and quality of care' proficiency 6.9 requires the graduate nurse to: *work with people, their families, carers and colleagues to develop effective improvement strategies for quality and safety, sharing feedback and learning from positive outcomes and experiences, mistakes and adverse outcomes and experiences.* As such 'effective improvement strategies' are changes made in real time, they are entrepreneurial, or more correctly intrapreneurial, solutions to day-to-day problems seen in the clinical setting. Nurses are, therefore, required to be equipped with many of the skills needed to be entrepreneurs, but often we fail to recognise them.

To understand the influence of entrepreneurism on the concept of intrapreneurism, we need to consider its antecedents. There is no commonly accepted definition of the terms 'entrepreneur' and 'entrepreneurship' and, furthermore, the meaning is shifting as it is applied to healthcare endeavours as intrapreneurism. In business or commercial terms an entrepreneur is someone who has a new idea and wishes to undertake a new venture with a responsibility for both the risks that may result and the outcome. There is an implicit sense that the entrepreneur will personally gain from the venture. Entrepreneurs will see opportunities for developments and take advantage of those opportunities; they can act as a catalyst for change and research and innovation, by introducing new technologies, increasing efficiency and productivity, and generating new products or services. An intrapreneur will essentially do the same but within the confines of an organisation. They will benefit less from the outcomes, but will be exposed to less attendant risk.

Neergård (2020) reported on a systematic review of the literature regarding nursing entrepreneurs and intrapreneurs. Neergård identified papers on nurse entrepreneurs in 16 countries with nurses specialising in primary care or secondary care as well as nurse entrepreneurs whose businesses do not deliver care as such. Some nurse entrepreneurs run businesses that support a small number of employees. Entrepreneurial nurses are identified as those who identify opportunities, generate ideas, use resources and start projects using their own initiative.

Neergård (2020) identifies barriers to entrepreneurial activity as including conflicts about mixing caring with business, finance and a general lack of entrepreneurial skill sets among nurses. The key drivers for nurse entrepreneurs, Neergård found, include the desire to affect change and quality improvement, professional identity, control over their working lives and an increased sense of being autonomous.

Activity 7.9   Skills development

Think of an area of practice, service delivery or patient care that you would like to see improved. Imagine you are going to present this idea to a *Dragons' Den*-type panel of peers. (If you are not familiar with the television programme *Dragons' Den*, look it up.)

1. Who would you have on the panel? What skills and knowledge would you expect them to have to make a decision about your idea?
2. Design a simple presentation that 'sells' your idea to the panel.

Hint

Go to the BBC web page **http://news.bbc.co.uk/1/hi/business/2943252.stm**, for tips on writing a business plan.

As this answer is based on your own research and reflections, there is no specimen answer at the end of the chapter.

The debate is still open on whether or not entrepreneurialism can drive forward a culture of innovation and creativity, benefiting patient care. There remain several obstacles, such as the prevailing ideology of the NHS as a public-sector organisation and therefore by default a 'not-for-profit industry', and the socialisation of nursing in its many forms that does not include a business frame of reference.

Chapter summary

In this chapter we have examined different organisational structures that you can map out in your own organisation. You can then identify where the decisions are made in your organisation which will, in turn, help you understand where to find information about the decisions. Nurses are playing an increasingly pivotal role in organisational decisions as government policy recognises they can not only represent their profession but also the patient's point of view. We have studied the governance requirements for NHS, and other healthcare, institutions to ensure they are meeting the standards required. We have identified what can happen when governance within an organisation does not serve or protect service users. While looking at standards, we considered how to improve care on a personal level through performance appraisal and compared some of the methods that can be used.

The chapter has also looked at the theory underpinning change management and contemporary theory developments. Change management is a huge subject and we have only briefly touched on the change-planning process to raise your awareness of the methods available. Finally, we looked at the potential for a newer approach to introducing change and improving standards, with an emphasis on social enterprise and entrepreneurial skills.

Activities: Brief outline answers

Activity 7.6 Reflection and critical thinking (p141)

1. Preparation for assessment and appraisal is the best method of ensuring levels of anxiety are minimised on the part of both the appraisee and the appraiser. This means ensuring the method and purpose of the process are clearly articulated and agreed beforehand, standards are transparent and evident in the organisation's policies, strengths as well as weaknesses are explored and the paperwork is available and prepared in advance by both parties. Further support for conducting appraisals can be found on the CIPD website listed in the useful websites section below.

Further reading

Barr, J and Dowding, L (2019) *Leadership in Healthcare*. London: Sage.

See Chapter 14: leadership for change.

Gopee, N and Galloway, J (2017) *Leadership and Management in Healthcare* (3rd edition). London: Sage.

See Chapter 6, Managing Change in Practice Settings.

Johnson, S (1999) *Who Moved My Cheese? An Amazing Way to Deal with Change in Your Work and in Your Life*. London: Vermilion.

An unusual but helpful look at change through the telling of a story.

Marquis, BL and Huston, CJ (2020) *Leadership Roles and Management Functions in Nursing: Theory and Applications* (10th edition). Philadelphia, PA: Wolters Kluwer Health.

See chapter 24, Performance Appraisal.

Jackson, C and Ellis, P (2010) Creative thinking for whole systems working, in Standing, M (ed) (2010) *Clinical Judgement and Decision-Making in Nursing: Theory and Practice* (pp 54–79). Milton Keynes: Open University Press.

Chapter 3, on complex systems theory.

Yoder-Wise, PS (2019) *Leading and Managing in Nursing* (7th edition). St Louis, MO: Mosby Elsevier.

See especially Chapter 18: Leading Change.

Useful websites

www.businessballs.com/change-management/

A good overview of change, change tools and the impact of change.

www.cipd.co.uk/hr-resources/factsheets/performance-appraisal.aspx

CIPD: Performance reviews. Understand the basics of performance reviews and how to ensure the process adds value to the organisation.

www.learnmanagement2.com

Organisation structures: The Learn Management website gives lots of theory and useful explanatory diagrams.

www.scottlondon.com/interviews/wheatley.html

The New Science of Leadership: an interview with Margaret Wheatley by Scott London.

www.healthcareimprovementscotland.org/our_work/patient_safety/tissue_viability_resources/plan_do_study_act_pdsa.aspx

The PDSA cycle page on Health Improvement Scotland's webpages.

www.bbc.co.uk/programmes/p00548f6

Chaos theory: BBC broadcast of radio programme chaired by Melvyn Bragg in 2002 with Susan Greenfield, Senior Research Fellow, Lincoln College, Oxford University, David Papineau, Professor of the Philosophy of Science, King's College, London and Neil Johnson, University Lecturer in Physics at Oxford University, discussing chaos theory. The broadcast explains chaos theory and its roots and application to modern-day usage. You will need Real Player software to listen to the broadcast, which lasts for 45 minutes.

www.youtube.com/watch?v=ZxuwVqyyrmM

Wendy Miles, entrepreneurial nurse 'Nurse Joey': Example of a nurse entrepreneur success that has improved nurses' working lives, benefited the organisation and released time for patient care. Wendy developed a handy pocket-like pouch to assist nurses; it saves time for nurses to carry small essential equipment about with them while they work.

www.entreprenurses.net

A website for UK nurses wishing to learn more about developing entrepreneurial skills and links to short learning modules, podcasts and relevant literature.

Chapter 8 Creating a learning environment

(Continued)

5.8 support and supervise students in the delivery of nursing care, promoting reflection and providing constructive feedback, and evaluating and documenting their performance.

5.9 demonstrate the ability to challenge and provide constructive feedback about care delivered by others in the team, and support them to identify and agree individual learning needs.

5.10 contribute to supervision and team reflection activities to promote improvements in practice and services.

Chapter aims

After reading this chapter you will be able to:

- identify what a learning environment is;
- explain why a learning environment is important;
- discuss how a learning environment might be created;
- consider your role in developing a learning environment.

Introduction

Nursing, in common with all health and social care, is evolving. In great part this evolution is driven by the society and culture we live in and by the changing technology we work with, developing understandings of the nature and experience of care. More recently, changes in health and social care have been driven by the need to respond to new and emerging threats to health, both at a local level and worldwide. Within this changing environment, there is a need for nursing to keep pace with developments. The increased professionalisation of nursing, clearly demonstrated by the move to an all-graduate profession, further requires nurses to be engaged with their own development and learning to meet the demands of twenty-first-century care provision. As can be seen in the descriptor for Platform 5, each nurse has the responsibility to act as *a role model for best practice in the delivery of nursing care*. This can only be achieved if we stay up to date with the latest learning and understanding.

Learning and developing are therefore constant and enduring requirements for all nurses, and the need to facilitate this is a key function of nurse leaders and managers. This chapter describes how the creation and maintenance of a learning environment in the clinical setting can contribute to the development of nurses and nursing. You will be challenged within this chapter to consider what this means for you as an individual, as well as how you might take the messages contained in it forward in your career as a leader or manager of nurses; that is, in the development of others. It is important to remember that your orientation to learning and the generation of learning environments have a direct, positive impact on patient care. In this respect, environments of care which are 'learning environments' allow us to express some of the values of care we discussed in detail in Chapter 1.

What are 'environments of care'?

Before we go on to consider what is meant by a 'learning environment', let's take a moment to consider what is meant by the term 'environments' in the sense used here. Environments refer to many things, including the physical nature of a building and its surroundings, as well as the meanings different people attach to the same physical space.

Activity 8.1   Reflection

To understand the ways in which different people attach different meanings to spaces, let's begin by reflecting on the nature of the work environment. When you are working in the hospital setting, consider the different ways in which people may experience the area in which you work. Consider how you experience the area, how the permanent staff experience it, how visiting staff experience it, how patients experience it and how visitors experience it. What are their different interpretations based on? Why is this important?

If you do not work in the hospital setting, consider the same questions in the context of the area in which you do work.

There are some possible answers and thoughts at the end of the chapter.

The interpretation of what an environment is, using the answers to the reflection, very much hinges on the function of the area concerned and your role in relation to that function. Different people experience the same area in quite different ways and have different views about the nature and workings of the same place. This is true both for people using an area for different purposes as well as for people who have a shared purpose or role with an area. For example, any nurse will have a unique experience of a place of work, shaped by their previous experiences as well as their experience of working in an area. This gives us some clues as to what an environment of care is about, but this is not the whole story.

Environments, especially care environments, are not only the product of what goes on there, but also of how people behave and interact. In this sense, environments can be considered to reflect the psychosocial nature of a place. Many commentators, most notably Charles Handy (1994), refer to environments as *cultures*, and in many ways this term is as useful as environments, if not more so. The word culture conjures up an image of something more ingrained, natural and all-encompassing than the term environment. In this sense a culture is not about nationality, race or ethnicity; it is about a shared sense of the psychosocial nature, *the feel,* of a place. This nature of the place is, therefore, a product of the human interaction and activity which happens there.

The psychosocial feel of a ward, clinical area or team is closely related to the ways in which the people there talk about, and to, each other, and the way in which they inter-act with people who are visitors to the area – the general ambience, if you like. In many respects, the environment or culture (we use the terms interchangeably) created in a care area reflects the *values* of the people who work there.

As nurses, and especially as leaders or managers, we can affect the environment in which we work. Understanding the impact we have as individuals and as leaders and managers is essential to understanding how to manage environments; you may find it useful to revisit the Johari window discussed in Chapter 1 at this stage to remind your-self about how others see us and how we see ourselves and what impact this has on relationships. The important aspect of the Johari window for the manager is how we manage the elements of the window which are shared with others; the open area, in which we allow others to see who we are. It is people's interpretation of who we are and how we behave that sets the tone for the wider team.

As a leader of people, the tone and nature of your interactions with others will set the benchmark by which others act. If you are seen not to care about where you work, or the people who work there, neither will the team. If you are brash, loud or condescending, then members of the team will be too. It is almost impossible to over-estimate the impact that leaders have on their immediate environment. The message about the impact of leaders on the environment of the team they lead is therefore clear – in most instances leaders create the culture.

Activity 8.2   Reflection

Think back on your placements; which teams were happy teams and which teams were not? Consider the values that were shared by the team, the way the manager spoke to people, how the trained nurses spoke to the students and support workers. Whose behaviours set the tone for the team? How and why did this happen? Thinking forward, what messages will you take from this about how you will act when you are a practice supervisor, mentor or team leader?

As this is based on your own observations, there is no specimen answer at the end of the chapter.

The Interprofessional CPD and Lifelong Learning UK Working Group (2019), which includes representative organisations from many health and social care professional bodies, state in their principles for continuing professional development and lifelong learning (p6) that *CPD and lifelong learning should:*

- *be each person's responsibility and be made possible and supported by your employer*
- *benefit service users*
- *improve the quality of service delivery*
- *be balanced and relevant to each person's area of practice or employment*
- *be recorded and show the effect on each person's area of practice.*

They define lifelong learning as: *Formal and informal learning opportunities that allow you to continuously develop and improve the knowledge and skills you need for employment and personal fulfilment* (p4).

With the advent of revalidation for nurses, all nurses need both to engage with and to record their continuing professional development activities (NMC, 2017). These activities contribute to the proof nurses require to demonstrate their practice is contemporaneous, informed by the current state of knowledge.

The role of the manager and leader in developing environments of care that support such learning development is critical. Creating a learning culture is something leaders must do by setting an example, not only in undertaking formal education themselves, but by learning from their team, their clients, from complaints and from their own practice (see the definition of lifelong learning above). The action of learning from others is an example of the exercise of the value of being 'other-regarding'. Being alert to sources of information as well as having the disposition to continually engage in learning with others is described in Chapter 1 of *Evidence Based Practice in Nursing* (Ellis, 2019b). In the model of evidence-based nursing described there, patient-centredness relies on the nurse being open to continual learning and development. The same is true of the leader who, in acting in this way, also acts as a role model to their team.

Learning from and with others is also a requirement of revalidation in that nurses have to demonstrate that they have gained practice-related feedback, written reflective accounts based on practice, and undertaken a reflective discussion with a peer (NMC, 2017). In following the template set out for revalidation by the NMC, the aspiring leader or manager can show how they demonstrate lifelong learning to the team.

In their systematic review, Qalehsari et al. (2017) identify the need for learning management and a suitable environment for learning as fundamental to the success of any lifelong learning strategy. The key message here is that, for a team to develop a learning culture, the leader or manager must take the lead in that learning, by role modelling learning behaviour and creating an environment where learning can be allowed to flourish.

What a learning environment is

A learning environment is essentially a set of attitudes, values and their corresponding actions that creates a culture in which learning and development can take place. Esterhuizen (2019, p29) identifies lifelong learning as being a valuable element of the continuing and continuous development of nursing professionals, and learning as being *multidimensional in terms of where and how it takes place.* The notion here is that the opportunities for learning and development that occur in the clinical setting are invaluable to the development of students. This point can be stretched further to include all the staff who work in a particular setting.

A ward, clinic or community team whose members are empowered to learn and develop will be able to provide meaningful care which not only reflects current clinical trends but also puts the patient at the heart of care. A team that operates in a learning environment will seize every opportunity to grow and develop and, as a result, their ability to care will be enhanced. A learning environment, then, is one that fosters positive development and change.

Curry et al. (2018) identify that organisational cultures have the power to accelerate learning and development, including the adoption of evidence-based practice, which in turn drives up performance. This further supports the idea that learning is more than an optional extra within the team; it is fundamental to the development of all members of the team and their practice. As such, the creation, adoption and maintenance of a learning environment is a fundamental approach to addressing the standards and proficiencies for registered nurse education highlighted at the start of the chapter. What this means for you as an individual student or nurse will be discussed later in the chapter.

Why learning environments are important

Increasing emphasis is being placed on the benefits associated with work-based learning in today's health and social care provision. In some part, this is evidenced by the increase in the number and range of foundation degrees available, and in the increasing provision of workplace learning modules in post-registration and postgraduate continuing professional development programmes for health and social care professionals.

The emphasis on work-based learning has been described by Attenborough et al. (2019) as arising from the global need to generate healthcare workers for the skills gap between registered nurses and healthcare support workers. Think of it this way; someone who is trained to change a dressing will do just that, while someone who understands how to change a dressing and what to look for in the way of healing will both change the dressing and be aware of alternative ways of doing the dressing, what infection might look like and what the nutritional needs of the patient might be. This latter way of working is an example of the activity that takes place in a learning environment where care is constantly evolving. Care which is the best it can be allows the nurse to exercise the values of providing high-quality, holistic care and, in this sense at least, the generation of a learning environment is a fulfilment of nursing values.

Developing a learning environment in the workplace also has the potential to bring many benefits to the team and to the individuals within the team. A team established in a learning culture can rapidly adapt to change and develop new ways of working that are consistent with best practice. Staff who work in, and adopt the values of, a learning organisation both feel, and are, more empowered to do their job and therefore have the ability to be more effective at what they do.

This is not about learning and changing for learning and changing's sake, it is about the advancement of care. One of the key complaints from nurses in any setting is that there are constant changes taking place. In a learning culture, change is seen as the norm when that change advances practice and brings about improvements in patient care.

Activity 8.3 Reflection

Reflect on the times in the classroom setting when you have engaged with the conversation around whatever it is you were learning. How did your engagement in the debate around the topic affect your learning? Did your contribution have an impact on what you learned and how you felt about what you learned?

There are some possible answers and thoughts at the end of the chapter.

Your answers to the above reflection probably demonstrate that on the occasions you engaged in what was happening in the classroom you learned more, felt happier and were clearer about the subject matter. What is more important is that engaging in what is going on probably helped you to feel more involved, part of something if you like, as well as feeling you contributed to the learning and development of the group as a whole.

Certainly, the same ideas translate into the practice setting, where engaging in learning, rather than being the passive recipient of knowledge, will greatly affect the learning you are able to take from a situation. Consider this scenario.

Case study: The same practice supervisor

Paul is a student nurse in his first year of training. Paul has a placement in a nursing home and is not at all happy with it as there is not enough high-tech care going on. Paul comes into work each shift, as he knows he must, and goes through the motions of caring for the elderly residents. He washes and helps to feed patients, but does little in the way of

(Continued)

(Continued)

communication and does not attempt to understand the care needs of those he nurses. Paul's practice supervisor offers little in the way of teaching, support or advice to Paul. Overall, it is a pretty poor experience and Paul does little more than endure it.

Mary, also a first-year student, is placed in the same home as Paul. Mary is keen to understand the care she is giving and what it means for the residents. She, too, would prefer to work somewhere more exciting, but has decided to get what she can in the way of learning from her experience. Mary talks to the residents and asks them about their lives. She observes them closely when washing and dressing them and takes note of issues such as the development of dry skin, skin tears or signs of weight loss. Mary listens when residents explain their symptoms and makes mental notes to look things up when she is off duty. Mary asks questions of her practice supervisor and explores ideas and tries to understand the new experiences she is having. Mary's practice supervisor is the same person supervising Paul, but offers Mary different learning opportunities and looks for ways to enhance her learning experience. Mary quickly starts to enjoy her placement and learns a lot about good-quality, holistic nursing care provision.

This case study may reflect some of the experiences you have had either as a student or a practice supervisor. What is important to understand is that the learning opportunities for both Mary and Paul are the same. What makes the difference is their approach to learning. Mary adopts a positive and open approach to learning. You might say she embodies a learning culture in herself, and as a result she gets a lot from her experience. Paul, on the other hand, closes himself off to learning and therefore gets little from his placement.

The reward for Mary in adopting this positive approach to her own development is enjoyment of the placement and enhanced learning. It is clear her practice supervisor also gained something from supervising Mary and therefore sought opportunities to support her development. Again, this is all about attitude. Mary shows her practice supervisor that she is engaged and values the experience. The extra effort the practice supervisor makes for her is in recognition of this.

As well as the opportunities that arise for self-development, learning cultures bring other rewards to the team and the organisation at large. Consider again the case study above. In being more diligent about her care provision, and in seeking not only to provide care but to understand the care she is giving, Mary has the opportunity to identify and prevent some potential complications arising in the residents she cares for. Such proactive nursing will benefit Mary, her patients, the team and the wider organisation in reducing the development of complication rates.

From the perspective of the home manager, the constructive approach to learning Mary has adopted demonstrates benefits for the team in the creation of a positive environment. For the team leader or home manager, the fostering of a positive learning culture will benefit the team in helping with staff recruitment and retention as well as the potential reduction in absences from work.

What is fascinating about this is the impact that allowing people to ask and answer questions can have on both morale and clinical outcomes. It seems such an insignificant thing to do, but clearly the effect is great.

Case study: Being alert to learning opportunities

Felicity was working with her practice supervisor Maxine, caring for Mr King. While helping Mr King to transfer from his bed to a chair, Felicity noticed him wincing but thought very little of it. Maxine had also noticed Mr King wincing and, unlike her supervisee, thought something was not right. Maxine went and checked Mr King's notes to be sure she understood his condition; she then asked Felicity to accompany her while they asked Mr King what it was that made him wince. Mr King said that it was when Felicity had supported him near his armpit; she was not rough though. Maxine considered this for a moment and then, after gaining Mr King's consent, examined his axilla, where she found some swelling of his lymph nodes.

The swelling did not fit with Mr King's diagnosis, so Maxine reported her finding to the ward doctor. The doctors examined Mr King and after ordering a chest X-ray, were able to see that he had asbestosis, which had not been previously diagnosed.

What this real-life case study shows is that working in a learning environment and being alert to what is going on in it can be of benefit to everyone, but most especially to the patient. Felicity learned as a result of this episode to not ignore things she saw about her, but to adopt a questioning approach to care.

Elements of the learning environment

So far, we have identified a definition of a learning culture and explored some of the benefits for the individual, team and organisation. In order to understand better the notion of learning environments it is now worth exploring the elements that go toward creating and sustaining them.

Peter Senge (1990), one of the leading writers on learning organisations, identifies five key elements – he calls them disciplines – which need to be in place for a learning organisation to be generated and maintained.

The five disciplines needed to create a learning environment

1. Systems thinking – this is essentially the ability to see the bigger picture. Seeing the big picture is an important element of nursing and leadership because of the complex nature of caring for people. Jackson and Ellis (2010) argue that whole-systems thinking in complex environments requires us to: identify all of the components of the system (people) and their roles as well as the nature of the interrelationships between them; recognise that working in a whole system is beneficial; and understand the risks of whole-systems working. The idea is that we see the interconnectedness of what each component (individual) of the system does and work to maximise its input (in much the same way as we explored team working in Chapter 3 and when we explored systems theory in Chapter 7).

2. Personal mastery – this is about the commitment of the people in the system to self-development. Self-development in this sense is about realising our potential and striving to be the best that we can be through constant and consistent self-development – clearly this relates to the exercise of our personal values, as we explored in Chapter 1.

3. Mental models – this requires us to identify and acknowledge the values, issues and beliefs that prevent us from being all we can be. This process involves reflection on ourselves and our motivations and becoming open and receptive to new ideas and ways of working. This often requires a change in both personal and team cultures.

4. Building shared visions – for the leader or manager, this is about gaining consensus on the view of how things should be from all the members of the team. When the team can agree to a vision of how things should be, they can work consistently and supportively to achieve it. As well as understanding your values, as a leader you will need to understand and acknowledge the values of the team.

5. Team learning – this is the final and fundamental aspect of creating a learning culture. One person does not make a culture alone. Nursing involves the co-operative working of nurses and other care professionals. Learning together facilitates the creation of relationships which enable the wider team to work together more effectively.

(Adapted from Senge, 1990)

What Senge's model demonstrates is that the creation of learning cultures requires the ability to see how things fit together, personal commitment, a change in thinking, shared drive and a willingness to learn together. So some of the messages here are about us as individuals and others about us and the way we interact in, or lead, teams.

Senge (1996) further identifies that the first step on the road to becoming a learning team or organisation is a willingness to allow people of all levels to lead in different ways. This requirement points to the need for everyone within the learning environment to commit to the values and practice of learning together.

What this means for you

The teams that work within a learning environment are made up of many individuals. As we have discussed, to a great extent the culture of the team derives from the actions and values of the leader or manager. The message is therefore clear for the leader or manager who wants to create a learning culture: lead by example. But what if you are not the manager or leader? What do the messages of this chapter hold for you?

As with all aspects of leading and managing, the first port of call is self. We saw in Chapter 5 that to deal with conflict effectively you must first ensure you are not the problem. We saw in Chapter 1 that to be an effective leader you must first know yourself and what drives and motivates you. Similarly, if you want to develop into the sort of leader who can promote learning and development, you must first develop yourself. Such development is not all about learning new things and ideas: it is more about your attitude to learning and development – the exercise of your values. For the student nurse this may mean adopting a more proactive approach to learning. You have made an important first step in choosing to read books such as this. If you are a trained nurse, your attitude to your own continuing professional development is equally important.

For the manager, this might include learning and understanding the strengths and weaknesses of your team so that you can use the strengths and develop the weaknesses to the benefit of the individuals, team and the patients you care for. Again, this is also about being a role model, being ready and willing to learn, to adapt and to ask questions pertinent to what is going on around you.

Not only is your attitude to self-development important, so too is your attitude to the learning and development of others. Are you happy to share what you know? Do you support colleagues and friends who need to understand something you know already? Are you willing to listen to and learn from others, perhaps even those you consider to be your juniors? Are you comfortable asking questions?

Activity 8.4 Critical thinking

In order to develop as a nurse learner and contribute to the development of learning environments of care, it is important you understand your journey as a nurse. To understand better what you need to do to develop, you must first reflect on your learning journey so far. Write a short biography of your learning as a person and a nurse to date: what have you learned, where have you learned it and how what you have learned has changed you. You should write this as if you are explaining who you are to someone meeting you for the first time.

As this is based on your own observations, there is no specimen answer at the end of the chapter.

There are some key challenges here about the way in which you present yourself to others as well as understanding what truly motivates you and your practice. There are multiple influences on what and how we learn; reflecting on these may start to tell us something about the type of environment we might want to create to promote learning. Certainly, the culture of the place in which you work now will impact on how you answer Activity 8.4 as well as how you feel about learning. Once again, the onus rests with you: how will you react to new learning opportunities? For the leader, the message about leading by example is clear: if you are comfortable about asking questions and developing your learning, your staff will be too; if you make people feel valued when they ask questions, they will ask them, and with questioning will come learning and development.

A word of caution here: leaders who are not serious about learning and developing with their staff create cultures which are the very antithesis on learning cultures. Such cultures are impoverished, they do not support development, they engage in outdated and outmoded practices, and good staff leave.

Developing a learning environment: The challenge

Now we have some understanding of the nature of learning environments, their benefits to the individual, team and wider organisation, the challenge is to understand for ourselves how we might create and develop such an environment. For the remainder of this chapter, this challenge takes the form of a series of activities to help you identify your orientation to learning environments, your experience of learning environments to date, and your understanding of how a learning environment might be created.

It is important that you explore these issues to address the requirement of the 2018 NMC *Future Nurse: Standards of Proficiency for Registered Nurses*. Platform 5 'Leading and managing nursing care and working in teams':

5.7 demonstrate the ability to monitor and evaluate the quality of care delivered by others in the team and lay carers.

5.8 support and supervise students in the delivery of nursing care, promoting reflection and providing constructive feedback, and evaluating and documenting their performance.

5.10 contribute to supervision and team reflection activities to promote improvements in practice and services.

Activity 8.5   Reflection

Reflecting on how you feel about learning in general, and learning within the practice setting in particular, will say something about your orientation to learning environments. Consider these questions and answer truthfully. You may find that some of the comments from practice supervisors in your practice assessment document will help you to identify how others perceive your learning behaviours: you might also like to reflect on the learning biography you wrote in Activity 8.3.

- How do you feel about new situations in the practice setting?
- Do you like new experiences or are you only comfortable with things that you know?
- How do you feel about asking questions?
- Does it matter who you are asking the questions of?
- Are you comfortable asking questions in front of others? Do you feel able to engage in learning with other professions?
- When a patient asks you a question to which you don't know the answer, do you make up an answer, say you don't know and find someone else, or tell the patient that you will find out?
- When you come across something that you do not understand, do you ignore it, ask questions of people who do, go away and look it up for yourself, ask questions and look it up?

As this is based on your own observations, there is no specimen answer at the end of the chapter.

What these questions will help you appreciate are the things you value in the way of learning and understanding in the clinical setting. While there are no wrong answers as such, primarily because these questions do not ask you what is the right thing to do but ask you what it is *you* do, there are some states of behaviour and responses which are perhaps more in line with the values needed to engage in a learning environment. An important issue covered in these questions is whether you are happy engaging in learning with other professionals.

Interprofessional learning and development has an interesting, if somewhat mixed, history in healthcare. Sanko et al. (2020), in their study of the perceived benefits of interprofessional education (IPE) involving nursing and medical students, identified how the students perceived IPE as benefiting their education because they learned to understand the importance of the work other professions undertake, they learned to understand where their colleagues' knowledge was better than theirs and they started to identify deficits in their own knowledge. The willingness and ability to engage in IPE therefore has benefits both for you as a nurse and, arguably, in enhancing person-centred care (Merriman et al., 2020).

What is needed from you, in terms of engaging in self-development which makes you fit for lifelong learning and engagement in, and potentially future creation of, learning environments, is: keenness to engage with and understand new situations and ways of working; a willingness to admit when you do not know something; a willingness to ask questions; and a desire to increase your understanding and the understanding of others when you are in a position to do so.

When we fail to embrace these key values as individual nurses, or nursing students, we do not fail ourselves alone, but also the wider team, organisation and ultimately our patients.

Activity 8.6   Critical thinking

Your orientation to learning environments will influence your understanding and feelings about learning environments. Think about how the environments in the various clinical areas that you have worked in have affected your learning. Consider how you have responded to the various learning opportunities presented to you:

- What have you done when the learning opportunities appear poor?
- Do you ask questions?
- Do you try to supplement this with your own reading and finding out?
- When faced with a poor learning environment, do you try to help more junior staff or students with their learning?
- What factors in the ward environment affect the learning opportunities available?
- Can you identify personal or group behaviours that appear to make a difference?

As this is based on your own observations, there is no specimen answer at the end of the chapter.

The questions in this activity point to the role you might play in creating your own learning opportunities, regardless of the culture of the place in which you are working. They ask questions about whether you role model positive learning behaviours and take a proactive stance in your own learning and that of others. The sort of person you choose to be in this respect will stay with you for much of your working life; it is often as students that we establish the blueprint for how we will act once qualified. This is the point of this chapter: developing the values of being inquisitive, seeking out knowledge and development while supporting the same opportunities in others as students prepares you for your role as a practice supervisor, team leader, team manager and creator of environments.

You are also asked to reflect on individual and group behaviours which impact on your learning and that of others in the area. Reflecting on and being aware of the behaviours and attitudes that promote, or hinder, learning, equip you with ideas about how you might behave in order to promote a positive learning environment. When you see good practice, you might choose to mirror it when you are a leader or manager; when you see poor practice, or practices which do not work well, you learn from these and do not repeat the same mistakes when you are in a position of influence.

Activity 8.7   Critical thinking

Given your orientation to learning environments and your experience of them to date, consider how you might go about creating a learning environment in the clinical setting if you were the manager:

- What strategies might you use to promote the change?
- How will you sell the idea to others?
- What strategies for learning might you promote to others?

The project management template below might help you plan your answer to this activity in a constructive manner.

Project management template
What is the purpose of the project? What do we do now and what is it we are trying to achieve?
Who is responsible for which aspect of the project? What skills and resources do we have available to us?
Who are our stakeholders? Who will this project affect and how will we get people on board with the idea?
How will we make a start? What do we need to do to start the change process?
What are the possible outcomes, both positive and negative? Consider here personal, team, organisational and patients.
What things might hinder the project and what might help it progress? What are the personnel and financial costs attached?
What should we have achieved by when and how will we know we have achieved these goals?
What will this look like when it is implemented? How will we know we have achieved our ultimate goals?
How and how often will we audit what we have done and maintain impetus, assuming we achieve our goals? What measure, both direct and indirect, might there be of our success?

As this is based on your own observations, there is no specimen answer at the end of the chapter.

The purpose of this activity is to demonstrate the thinking, planning, communicating and team working that need to go into the initiation of a change project. Committing to becoming more learning-oriented for yourself and developing a learning culture in a team require commitment, time, effort and good communication – and role modelling.

By working through the template you should now be more familiar with the sorts of processes required to make such an important change.

Learning environments and values

This book identifies how we can develop as managers and leaders who exercise the values which brought us into nursing in the first place. As we have seen throughout the book, there are many values that we need to exercise as leaders of care. As we saw in Chapter 2, the most famous current example of these values is Cummings' (2012) 6 Cs: care, compassion, competence, communication, courage and commitment.

The development of a learning environment that is underpinned by the values of good care, compassion and communication requires us as leaders to exercise courage and commitment in developing ourselves to become more competent at what we do and in supporting the developing competency of others. In this sense we can see that learning environments contribute strongly to enabling nurses to express their values.

Chapter summary

In this chapter we have seen that environments or cultures of care are important in the functioning of health and social care teams. We have identified that learning cultures are important for the sustained development of nursing teams and the wider healthcare system. We have identified that for learning cultures to succeed there is a need for engagement of all the members of the team. The role of the individual leader, nurse or nursing student within the team has been identified as being fundamental to the success of any culture.

We have also seen how developing learning environments serves to develop environments in which nursing values, as embodied in the 6 Cs, can thrive, to the benefits of staff, individual nurses and, most importantly, patients.

The challenge that has been presented in this chapter has been one of engaging in self-development as a learner for yourself before considering taking on the extended task of creating a learning environment in your place of work as you develop through to a position of leadership.

Activities: Brief outline answers

Activity 8.1 Reflection (p155)

As a student transiting through an area as part of your training, you may see the area as a place of learning while having a feeling of being an outsider. Permanent staff may be comfortable with the area and regard it very much as a place of work. Visiting staff, such as physiotherapists and social workers, may experience the area as an extension of a bigger area of work. Patients may experience the environment as one in which they do not belong and as somewhere they can at least leave.

When working in the community, your place of work is often someone else's home, a place where you are both at work and a visitor, and where your patient is both patient and home owner.

Activity 8.3 Reflection (p159)

When we engage in open conversation about a topic, we become involved. Being involved in something brings a sense of belonging and worth. This sense of worth helps us to understand our place in contributing to something bigger than ourselves, in this case the collective understanding of the topic. This reflects nicely the concept of the learning environment, where people feel they belong because they are not only learning together, they are also contributing to that learning.

Further reading

Buchanan, D and Huczynski, A (2019) *Organizational Behaviour* (10th edition). Oxford: Pearson.

A well-known and widely referred to textbook which explains elements of how organisations work.

Handy, C (1994) *Understanding Organizations.* London: Penguin.

A great and classic text on organisational cultures.

Luhman, JT and Cunliffe, AL (2013) *Key Concepts in Organization Theory.* London: Sage.

An easy to read primer all about organisations.

Mullins, LJ (2019) *Essentials of Organisational Behaviour* (12th edition). London: Oxford: Pearson.

A comprehensive guide to understanding organisations.

Useful websites

www.cipd.co.uk/knowledge/culture/working-environment

An interesting selection of resources about workplace cultures from the CIPD.

www.investorsinpeople.com/knowledge/

A useful website with many resources including ones about culture. Register for access to the guides, including some on employee engagement.

Chapter 9 Developing confidence as a manager and leader

5.6   exhibit leadership potential by demonstrating an ability to guide, support and motivate individuals and interact confidently with other members of the care team.

5.7   demonstrate the ability to monitor and evaluate the quality of care delivered by others
in the team and lay carers.

Platform 6: Improving safety and quality of care

Registered nurses make a key contribution to the continuous monitoring and quality
improvement of care and treatment in order to enhance health outcomes and people's
experience of nursing and related care. They assess risks to safety or experience and take
appropriate action to manage those, putting the best interests, needs and preferences of
people first.

At the point of registration, the registered nurse will be able to:

6.1   understand and apply the principles of health and safety legislation and regulations
and maintain safe work and care environments.

6.2   understand the relationship between safe staffing levels, appropriate skills mix, safety
and quality of care, recognising risks to public protection and quality of care, escalating concerns appropriately.

6.4   demonstrate an understanding of the principles of improvement methodologies,
participate in all stages of audit activity and identify appropriate quality improvement strategies.

Chapter aims

After reading this chapter you will be able to:

* discuss the practice–leadership continuum;
* demonstrate an awareness of some of the issues with transition to leadership and management roles;
* discuss some of the key challenges that face new leaders and managers;
* explain how confidence might be developed in the new manager.

Introduction

Throughout this book we have introduced you to ideas and theories about leadership
and management, and some of the tasks leaders and managers undertake. You will
have noted that many of the tasks of management start with understanding yourself
and your orientation to a situation, role or task, as well as having a clear appreciation of
your values and those of the organisation in which you work.

This chapter will look at some of the issues facing the new leader or manager, identifying and focusing on some strategies that might be used to help develop ability and confidence. Other issues that commonly confront new managers will also be addressed, with some ideas about how these might be managed. As with all the chapters in this book it is important you engage with the activities, as they represent tools for self-development that may help to enhance your learning and development as a manager as well as your confidence to lead.

The transition to leadership

When you first thought about being a nurse and when you were interviewed for your nurse training, it is likely you thought and talked about all the ways you could help people as a practising nurse. As you progress through your training and into your nursing career you may start to aspire to leadership and management, seeing this as a way of extending the scope of what you can do for and with patients.

It is worth reflecting here on the different stages of professional life we adopt as we move from practising nurse through to leadership and management roles. Causer and Exworthy (2003) classically identify six stages on the path from practice to management which they regard as being stages on a continuum.

Roles within the professional–management continuum

1. The practising professional: The main task of the practising professional is the provision of care. Within this definition there are two groups of people:

    (a) the pure practitioner – who undertakes professional roles but has no supervisory role;

    (b) the quasi-managerial practitioner – who undertakes a professional caring role, and has some responsibility for supervising others or allocating resources.

2. The managing professional: The main function of these professionally trained managers is the supervision of other professionals and the allocation and management of resources. Again, this group is split into two groups:

    (a) the practising managing professional – who still works in the delivery of care as well as managing others and resources;

    (b) the non-practising managing professional – who does not deliver care, but supervises other professionals and manages resources.

3. General managers: These are managers who manage others who are involved in the delivery of professional care, but not at the day-to-day (**operational**) level. Again, these are subdivided into two categories:

(a) non-professionally grounded general managers – who are not part of the profession they are managing;

(b) professionally grounded general managers – who are part of the profession they are managing.

(Adapted from Causer and Exworthy, 2003)

What Causer and Exworthy (2003) identify is that the transition from being a practitioner to being a manager can be subtle and occurs in stages. The move from practice to management is therefore not a stark one, whereby one day you are a nurse practising on the ward and the next day you are a general manager. The process identified here will most certainly allow for some adaptation and personal and professional development to take place. This notion links well with the ideas around being an individual within a learning organisation, identified in Chapter 8.

Activity 9.1   Critical thinking

Taking the categories of professionals and managers that Causer and Exworthy identify, consider all the people who work in the team in the clinical area in your most recent placement. Which of the roles identified in the model do they fit into, if any? What characteristics of Causer and Exworthy's descriptions do they display? What was their previous role? You may want to take this activity a step further and discuss the changing nature of the individual roles with them.

As this is based on your own observations, there is no specimen answer at the end of the chapter.

Undertaking this activity will help you discover there are layers of responsibility, leadership and management in the clinical setting. The degree of certainty people have in the roles they undertake can grow and develop as they move from one position to another, and as they learn from their own practice and from those around them. What is important in the transition from practice to management remains the focus on the values which you came into nursing with (see Chapter 1) and a willingness to develop both yourself and others around you (see Chapter 8).

Self-esteem and transition

As with all development, the changes that need to occur for you to move from school, or from another job, to becoming a nursing student, to qualifying and beyond, require some psychological adjustment. Even when we are excited about something, there are adjustments to make to the ways in which we think and behave as we move on to something new. Sometimes the adjustments are in response to whatever it was we aspired to not quite living up to what we expected from it. Either way, it is worth considering the nature of change and transition from being a practising nurse to being a leader.

> ## Activity 9.2   Reflection
>
> Think about how you felt during your first few weeks in a care environment. One day you were a member of the public and the next a carer or a student nurse. Taking responsibility for the welfare of other human beings requires some adjusting to; reflect on your feelings at this time and think about how you managed to cope with this transition.
>
> *There are some possible answers and thoughts at the end of the chapter.*

Your answers to Activity 9.2 will show that emotions experienced during even a much wanted change can be quite overwhelming. What this tells us for planning to make the change from practitioner to leader or manager is that there are a host of normal emotions and responses to change we need to prepare for.

Perhaps the first lesson is that an emotional response to change is normal, so you should not be surprised if you are a little stressed by a promotion or being given a leadership role! It is worth pausing here to consider the nature of the emotional responses people have as they adapt and evolve.

Bridges and Bridges (2017), leading writers about the change process, remind us how things change, while people go through transitions. Transition involves loss and letting go, as well as developing a new understanding of how things are. In the case of a nurse making the transition from practising nurse to leader or manager, this involves a redefining of their professional and personal identity. Transition is not another word for change in this sense, it is a parallel process that people go through, some with the need for support. Bridges and Bridges' model of transition captures these ideas in a three-stage process.

Three-phase process of transition

1. Ending, losing, letting go: at this stage people have to make the adjustment to not being who they were before. For example, a student nurse on the point of qualifying must adjust to being qualified and accountable; or a staff nurse being promoted to junior sister may have to adapt to having more responsibility.

2. The neutral zone: at this stage people try to make sense of who they are now and how things are going to be. Student nurses start to accept they are now qualified and begin to adopt the persona of someone who is accountable; junior charge nurses start to understand they have to be the one to find solutions to problems and act as role models.

3. The new beginning: a new identity is forming and there is increased clarity about what is expected. There is a sense of urgency and of wanting to get on with the job.

New staff nurses start to feel confident in their own ability and what they are doing; the new charge nurse feels comfortable about being a role model and overseeing the work of the team.

(Adapted from Bridges and Bridges, 2017)

While progressing through transition – it is normal for people to experience a whole range of different emotions even if the change is something that is wanted. Understanding these emotions and recognising them in yourself, as well as others, is a good way of helping maintain and develop your confidence as you progress through your career. When these emotional responses feel overwhelming, it is worth harking back to our discussion of values in Chapter 1; what is important about the values of caring and of leading care is that they are the same values, the only difference is how they are expressed. You may find it useful here to revisit the case study from Chapter 1 (p7) in which Deirdre, the ward sister, explains to Julius, the newly qualified nurse, how what she does as the ward manager supports the ward staff in the delivery of care.

Hopson and Adams (1976) propose a useful, and enduring, model identifying some of the stages people go through when transitioning. This model is not linear (people move through it in different directions at different rates and may skip stages), nor does it necessarily apply to all transitions people go through; nevertheless, it is a useful model for helping us to understand the emotional response to transition.

Changes in self-esteem during transitions

- Immobilisation: the feeling of being unable to act and being overwhelmed. Transitions for which people are unprepared and ones associated with negative expectations may intensify this stage.
- Minimisation: a coping mechanism. People often deny the change is happening. This reaction is common in a crisis that is too difficult to face head-on.
- Depression: some people become depressed when facing the reality of change.
- Accepting reality: occurs when a person begins to let go of things and starts to accept the reality of the change.
- Testing: begins when the reality of the change has been accepted. At this stage people start to try out new behaviours to cope with the new situation.
- Seeking meaning: a reflective stage, during which people try to work out how things are different.
- Internalisation: the final stage of the process, during which the new situation becomes accepted. The new understanding then becomes part of the person's behaviour.

(Adapted from Hopson and Adams, 1976)

When making the transition from student to trained nurse and then on to leader and manager, it is useful for us to be aware of the ways in which we react to change as individuals. Being aware of our own responses enables us to make sense of, and progress through, the various emotional responses to change, as well as managing how we behave around and support other people.

Change and transition are not only confined to the workplace: changes in home circumstances, bereavement and ill health will all impact on how people feel and behave. Being aware of this and maintaining good channels of communication allow the leader or manager to develop skills and confidence in people management which are strongly associated with emotional intelligence. The emotionally literate manager is sensitive to the verbal and non-verbal cues given off by their staff rather than waiting to be told that someone is upset or stressed. They can anticipate an emotional response to change and are therefore ready to address it.

Activity 9.3   Evidence-based practice and research

Hopson and Adams' model of the changes in self-esteem during change is similar to a famous model of the stages of grief by Elizabeth Kubler-Ross. Go online and find the Kubler-Ross model and read what it says (see the useful websites at the end of the chapter). Compare and contrast what you learn about the stages of grief in this model with the Hopson and Adams model. What similarities and differences do you notice? What does this tell you about the psychological impact of change in the workplace?

There are some possible answers and thoughts at the end of the chapter.

Being prepared for the emotional response that you may have to a change in your role or work circumstances means you will be able to better prepare yourself mentally. As a leader or manager, providing support to your team through supervision, information giving and being supportive will mean you can help reduce some of the impact of negative emotional responses to transition.

Activity 9.4   Evidence-based practice and research

Look up the **Holmes–Rahe Life Event Rating Scale** (see the useful websites at the end of the chapter) and read the categories of change people find most stressful; some of the listed changes may surprise you.

As this is based on your own observations, there is no specimen answer at the end of the chapter.

Developing yourself as a leader

This section will present and examine some of the strategies you can use to prepare yourself for a leadership or management role while managing your emotional response to change. All the ideas presented here are tools and tactics that can be used while you are a student, staff nurse, charge nurse or beyond to improve and enhance your own confidence, understand yourself better and develop self-discipline.

Robinson-Walker (2020, pviii) says *self mastery is a continuous journey toward excellence, one that can be undertaken by nurses at any stage of their nursing and leadership careers.* The thing is, only you can truly know whether you are willing to put effort into your self-mastery and development.

Set incremental goals

Target setting is a key factor in self-motivation. If you cannot be bothered to put in the work, then whatever it is you are aiming to do will not happen. Motivation is an interesting tool, in personal, professional and leadership development. Herzberg (1959), the most famous theorist in this area, proposed the motivation–hygiene theory of job satisfaction. In essence, Herzberg's theory suggests people will work hard to achieve the hygiene factors, as achieving these will make them happy, but only for a short time. It is only the true motivators that keep people happy and motivate them in the longer term.

Motivation–hygiene theory of job satisfaction

Hygiene factors

- quality of relationships with supervisors;
- working conditions;
- salary;
- status;
- job security;
- quality of relationship with subordinates;
- personal life.

True motivators

- achievement;
- recognition;
- opportunity for advancement;
- work itself;
- responsibility;
- sense of personal growth.

(Adapted from Herzberg, 1959)

What we can see is that motivation lies in taking responsibility and improving on what we do and therefore who we are. For the student this may mean getting better at writing essays, by learning from feedback. For the leader it may be important to ensure the hygiene factors are all in place before worrying too much about the motivators, although some things remain outside the sphere of influence of most nurse leaders.

Case study: Recognising the value of motivation

Jacinta had recently been promoted to Modern Matron in the surgical care team. Jacinta had worked her way up through the team over a period of years and was very much aware of the issues that preoccupied the staff. She knew that staff morale was incredibly low as the team felt overworked, understaffed, poorly cared for and generally neglected. Jacinta understood the team felt the need for further professional development as well as some clarity about promotion opportunities. Jacinta was also aware that the whole team were fed up with the state of their coffee room, which had been allowed to deteriorate over time. She knew she needed to do something fast to raise the morale of the whole team and to consolidate her position as the team leader, but she also knew she had limited funds with which to do anything.

Jacinta considered her options and decided there were some things she could do collectively for the team as well as some things she needed to do for individuals within the team to raise morale, gain trust and improve motivation. Jacinta decided to spend some of the capital budget available to her to buy new furniture for the coffee room. By doing so she improved working conditions for the whole team and addressed a hygiene need.

Jacinta quickly realised she could not provide the motivation the staff needed purely by spending money (which was not available to her anyway), so she identified new roles for various members of the team as link nurses for infection control, diabetes and wound management, providing some of the junior staff with a sense of increased responsibility, recognition and personal growth. Furthermore, Jacinta took it upon herself to try to make sure staff went home when their shifts ended. She praised effort and cultivated her relationships within the team, addressing key hygiene and motivational needs.

This case study, based on a real-life experience, demonstrates how easy it can be to grow as a leader or manager in the eyes of the team by making small but important changes which show the team the manager cares about them as individuals. As we saw in Chapter 2, demonstrating that you, as a leader, care about people is a key strategy for gaining the trust of the team.

Facilitating and bringing about the changes meant not only did the team feel happier, but Jacinta's confidence as a manager grew as she started to notice a change in the morale of the team and that the team had started to trust her as someone who both cared about them and was able to get things done.

Trust is an important element of the role of the manager, ensuring the work which the team needs to get done is done. In their meta-analysis, Dirks and Ferrin (2002) demonstrated how trust is important in the prevention and management of conflict; they also demonstrated how having a positive attitude as a leader will reflect in your orientation to work, the *manner* by which you achieve goals, and this in turn leads to another important observation, which is about citizenship.

Because the team learn to trust the way you work and the types of goals you set yourself, they start to feel responsibility toward the things you find important. This citizenship is, in essence, about the ways in which we behave toward each other and how we share some common values and aspirations. In turn, this means that the leader can be confident the members of the team will also work toward achieving the goals the leader has set, because they also want to.

Learn to actively listen

For the nurse as much as the leader or manager, listening is a fundamental skill. When we learn to listen to others, be it in a formal or informal situation, we can understand the true context of situations. Listening also enables us as nurses and as managers, to find solutions to problems that we may not have identified for ourselves.

Managing information was identified in Chapter 2 as one of Mintzberg's (1975) roles of the manager. Information allows us to make decisions that are well grounded, and learning to listen and to be enquiring will enhance your ability both to understand what is going on around you and to make sound decisions.

In this context, listening is more about taking the time to hear what people are saying, and trying to understand it, while placing what we are hearing in the context of what we know. As an active skill, listening is important for personal growth and professional development (Jackson and Ellis, 2010).

Activity 9.5   Evidence-based practice and research

Go online and find some websites that talk about the skills you need to become an active listener. Make a list of the skills and tips the websites identify and think about how they compare to how you are when you are listening to other people. Take the time to then practise some of the skills you identify when talking to friends, colleagues and patients.

As this is based on your own observations, there is no specimen answer at the end of the chapter.

Understand, then communicate

The aim of listening properly and effectively is to understand. Understanding situations and new ideas is a good way of developing your confidence. Part of understanding is the ability to ask the right questions at the right time, as well as being able to communicate your ideas in an effective way. Communicating effectively hinges on your ability to understand what other people know as well as what it is they want.

As a leader or manager your confidence will develop as people become aware you are able to communicate clearly. Clear communication will mean members of the team understand what it is you want from them; it allows you to explain ideas and delegate effectively. Learning to understand before speaking is a key skill for the aspiring leader or manager; we have all been in situations when individuals have made themselves look silly because they have said something that demonstrates they have not been listening.

Believe in yourself

Self-belief is not the same as arrogance or being egocentric. Self-belief is having the confidence you can do something well and doing it. Self-belief comes only from practice, from exercising your leadership muscles by developing and maintaining good relationships with staff and understanding yourself. When you believe in what you are doing as well as believe you can do it, other people will see this and feel able to follow your lead.

Leaders and managers who are confident in their own abilities are better able to develop their team and are comfortable with members of the team having better skills and knowledge in certain areas than they do. The manager who has self-belief will recognise the team is more important than self, and this team-focused attitude will help develop trust.

Don't be afraid to make mistakes

Making mistakes is part of life. This is as true for the leader or manager as it is for individual team workers. Learning to reflect enables us to make sense of what has happened as well as learning how to do something better in the future (see Esterhuizen, 2019). Learning from our mistakes can make us stronger as individuals and as leaders as we develop new ways of working which take account of what we have learned as well as where we want to be. Failure often precedes success, as it is through trying new ways of working that we can be innovative (Tian and Yue Wang, 2014).

Part of the process of growing as a person and a leader is the ability to accept responsibility for the things we get wrong. When, as leaders, we develop the ability to accept responsibility for our own actions, we can role model responsibility and accountability to our team.

Within the team context, supporting others who make mistakes empowers them to make decisions and take actions with the confidence they will be supported; a key element of trust. Bekirogullari (2019) reminds leaders that to achieve success they need to allow their team to try new things and make mistakes. So being brave enough to try new things and new ways of working is useful in developing your confidence in yourself and in your ability to lead others.

Learn to manage your time effectively

The pressures on time for leaders come in all shapes and forms and can quite easily disrupt the working day. Time management is the art of getting the most from your time by developing an awareness of what time is and how it is used. Understanding how to use time wisely will help you understand what you can achieve and in what time frame. This will translate into the confidence to take on new roles and tasks or allow you to explain why you cannot.

John Adair (1990), whose model of action-centred leadership we looked at in Chapter 2, suggests leaders and managers need to learn to manage time before they can manage anything else. He sees good time management as a requirement for allowing us to focus on what we do and achieving our goals. Time management is therefore about being focused on attaining goals and achieving results. In Adair's view, there are ten principles by which good time management can be achieved.

Theory summary: Adair's ten principles of good time management

1. Develop a personal sense of time: understand where your time goes, where it is wasted and where it could be better used. For the leader it may also uncover areas of work that might be better delegated to someone else.
2. Identify long-term goals: know what you want to achieve in life and work. Adair recognises values as being a key driving force behind setting such goals.
3. Make medium-term plans: understand what you need to do to prepare you to achieve your long-term goals and plan how to achieve them. Medium-term plans involve setting realistic goals that are measurable.
4. Plan the day: without planning what you will achieve today, you cannot know whether you have used your time wisely. Learn to say no to things that are a poor use of your time or which interfere with you achieving your goals.
5. Make the best use of your best time: understand what times of day you work best and work during them. Take time to think about issues and ideas that need planning while doing other more mundane activities.
6. Organise office work: make sure you organise your life and your working space so things you need are at hand when you need them.
7. Manage meetings: understand what you want from a meeting and stick to the time available for this.
8. Delegate effectively: consider what things you need to do and what might be better done by someone else.

(Continued)

(Continued)

9. Make use of committed time: plan to use time that is usually wasted waiting or travelling and use it to good effect, perhaps reading something, making phone calls, or thinking constructively about an issue.

10. Manage your health: things are easier to achieve when we are well, so look after yourself and make time to do things that are necessary for your physical and mental well-being.

(Adapted from Adair, 1990)

For Adair, making good use of time and being aware of what we can achieve in a given time frame are key to developing confidence and being successful. Knowing what you achieved and why is a great motivator.

Activity 9.6   Evidence-based practice and research

Keep a diary of all the things you do for one week. Split the time into 15-minute slots and record what you do: be careful to record wasted time as well as activities. After a week review the diary and identify times during which you could have done something useful if you were prepared. Consider how you might adapt some of your ways of working and habits to allow you to achieve more in the time available to you.

You may wish to use this exercise as a springboard for planning your personal development and planning what you want to achieve, how and by when. Understanding how you use time will enable you to plan this more effectively.

As this is based on your own observations, there is no specimen answer at the end of the chapter.

Once you understand how you use time and where you can fit in tasks to make your use of time more efficient, you will start to see that it is possible to fit more into your day. When you free up time you can decide how to use it, perhaps undertaking more work or engaging in a hobby or other interest.

Know your values

You may feel we have discussed values too much in this book; however, since our values shape the ways we behave, their importance cannot be overestimated. Knowing what your values are as a human, as a nurse and ultimately as a leader or manager, will mean there is consistency in the ways in which you act. Sticking to your values will not only mean you are happier in whatever you do; it will mean the team will know what to expect from you and, perhaps more importantly, what you expect from them. Trust, which is how leaders get things done, relies on leaders demonstrating their integrity to their followers (Setyaningram et al., 2020).

One of the issues that face nurses as they move from practice to leadership and management roles is their lack of clarity about their identity. It is easy to forget things that mattered to you as a student or staff nurse, the values that guided your desire to be a nurse and your subsequent practice as you become more engaged with leadership and management roles. Understanding what your values are now, and being able to discuss them in a meaningful way, will help you remain grounded and focused as you prepare for leadership.

Issues such as fairness, treating people as equals, being polite and behaving with care and compassion might feature on your list. These are all basic values that are easily forgotten in the milieu of the busy working day. Practising these values and ensuring they become part of who you are and how you act will allow you to establish a reputation as someone who knows what they are doing and what they are about. The NMC (2018a) *Future Nurse: Standards of Proficiency for Registered Nurses* document talks about the duty of the nurse to act as a role model to others in several places. This bears witness to the fact that, as a registered nurse, you must demonstrate not only the proficiencies, but also the positive behaviours the NMC and the public expect of you at all times.

Activity 9.7   Reflection

Take some time now to consider the things that you value as a human being and as a nurse. Think about what you might have said at interview about why you wanted to train as a nurse, or the skills and attributes that you bring to your current role. Consider the issues in practice that cause you frustration and the behaviours which you think are unacceptable from your colleagues. Write these things down and keep them safe. Spend some time over the next few weeks thinking about and observing these issues in practice and considering what you might do to change poor practice and role model good leadership values when you are able to do so.

As this is based on your own observations, there is no specimen answer at the end of the chapter.

It is all too simple when you become a leader to forget how it feels to be led, so instead of addressing and rejecting the negative leadership behaviours and values you have witnessed, you adopt the same negative leadership behaviours.

Develop resilience

One of the hallmarks of the strong leader or manager is the ability to be resilient. Resilience is the ability to take criticism constructively, listen to what people are saying about your organisation and team without taking it personally, and to understand the meaning of situations.

Resilience is not about developing a thick skin, not least because a thick skin prevents effective empathy. Resilience is more about having the ability to deal with stressful situations.

Here, again, it is important to understand yourself. If you understand what things you find stressful and why, you can learn to manage them.

Case study: Developing resilience

Loiselle was a newly qualified nurse on a general medical ward. She had not worked on the ward as a student and did not know any of the team. Loiselle found the healthcare support workers and nursing associates on the ward were very free and easy about making complaints, grumbling and suggesting how things might be done better.

As the new staff nurse, Loiselle was often the target of these suggestions and gripes. Loiselle found it hard to cope with all the information and after a few weeks in post started to take all the negative comments personally, as if they were a reflection on her. She started to feel incredibly stressed and did not want to go to work anymore. Loiselle discussed her feelings with the ward manager. The ward manager, who had come up through the ranks in the hospital, suggested to Loiselle that she stopped taking all the criticism as personal and that she turned issues back to the other staff, with questions like 'how would you see this progressing?' or 'what would you suggest we do to improve this?' The manager also suggested Loiselle should not accept some of the unfair things people were saying and that she should tell them that what they were saying was unfair. She reminded her the staff were 'testing her' because she was new.

Asking these simple questions reminded Loiselle that the problems were not hers. She started turning questions back to the team and reminded staff that if they had an issue with how things were, they should talk to the manager. She developed a reputation for being fair-minded and not someone who would tolerate unreasonable behaviour.

This case study demonstrates how one of the skills of being a leader is learning what a gripe or moan means and who it is aimed at. It also demonstrates how taking on board issues which are not personal, and are not purely your own problem, may lead to a sense of helplessness and futility. Taking charge of such situations by being brave enough to ask for a solution (rather than saying something like 'I know what you mean', try saying 'how might this be resolved?') can help you, as the leader, to develop delegation skills and demonstrate trust. It can also help you move away from being weak and downtrodden.

So in part, resilience is about developing strategies to deflect and reflect problems back to where they really belong; although, of course, this does not mean every problem that comes your way belongs to someone else!

Confront challenging situations

Developing resilience leads us into the next skill, which is about not being afraid to get involved. There are times as a nurse when situations arise and people behave in ways that we feel are not acceptable. Such situations need confronting, and learning to communicate your point in a way that links in with your expressed values is a good place to start. For a manager or leader, there is often nowhere to hide and learning to confront difficult situations early is a good idea. One strategy for the novice is to accompany more experienced staff who are, for example, breaking bad news; ask questions about what they did after the event and reflect on the answers. We discussed some strategies in Chapter 5 where we suggested some of the approaches to managing conflict might include: collaborating, compromising, accommodating, competing and dodging (Thomas and Kilmann, 1974). The art of good leadership lies in using a right approach for any given situation, and there is often more than one, and not becoming known for always using the same approach regardless of the nature of the situation that has arisen.

Another sort of challenging situation is one that you do not understand or about which you are uncertain. The key to developing the ability to confront such a situation is developing the confidence to ask questions. Not knowing is not a weakness, pretending you do might well be. Asking questions allows for understanding and should not be mistaken for weakness. As an aspiring leader it is important that you develop a reputation for being enquiring and that you support others in their efforts to achieve self-awareness and self-development.

Develop your emotional intelligence

Perhaps many of the ideas contained in this book can be boiled down to one key message: develop your emotional intelligence. Throughout the book we have suggested there is a need to understand yourself and the part you play in many situations before you look at what other people are doing or saying. You also need to understand where other people are coming from and what motivates their actions.

Emotional intelligence requires you to be able to use this understanding to communicate effectively. Emotional intelligence, as well as the ability and desire to help others achieve their goals, reflect strongly on many of the standards of proficiency for registered nurse education highlighted at the start of this chapter.

From your practice you will know that many of the skills, attributes and roles that nurses undertake require them to be self-aware and aware of the needs of others. This awareness, which you are required to develop as a student nurse, will most certainly be a big part of the suite of competencies that we have suggested in this book go toward creating effective managers and leaders. What is important for you as you develop from student nurse to staff nurse, sister and beyond is that you conscientiously continue to develop these capabilities in such a way that they become part of how you behave and, therefore, who you are. Nurse leaders and managers are entrusted with the management and leadership of people delivering care to some of the most vulnerable in society. By becoming a good role model, you can be more certain that the care you and your team deliver lives up to the lofty ideals of modern nursing practice.

Chapter summary

In this chapter we have explored the journey from student nurse to nurse manager and what this might mean for us in managing our emotional responses to change and transition. We have identified some important strategies, skills, tactics and values which, taken together, can better prepare you for the responsibilities leadership and management bring. We have demonstrated how developing trust can have a positive impact on the development of self and of the wider team. The challenge lies in engaging with these ways of being from the start of your career and nurturing them as you develop onward into your career as a nurse and a leader.

Activities: Brief outline answers

Activity 9.2 Reflection (p174)

The emotions people experience during changes and transitions are not purely tied to the sort of change they are experiencing. All change can bring fear and trepidation, even the changes that are wanted and exciting. The move into a caring role requires some thought about who you put first, how you behave, what impact the emotional investment will have on you as a person and how you will adapt.

Activity 9.3 Evidence-based practice and research (p176)

When you compare the model of the stages of grief with that of changes in self-esteem during transition you will notice they both evoke strong reactions. These reactions include not accepting what is happening through various stages of frustration and anger and finally to some sort of acceptance. Both models identify how people do not necessarily proceed through all the stages, nor necessarily in order and not to a set timeframe, and people can go backward as well as forward through the model.

For the leader this is potentially tricky as, at any one stage of a change, the staff involved can be at different stages in their reactions, while some staff who appeared to have moved might move backward.

Further reading

Davis, N (2011) *Learning Skills for Nursing Students.* Exeter: Learning Matters.

Gives helpful advice for gaining knowledge and confidence.

Esterhuizen, P (2019) *Reflective Practice in Nursing* (3rd edition). London: SAGE.

Essential advice on how to understand yourself and grow in professionalism.

Forde-Johnson, C (2018) *How to Thrive as a Newly Qualified Nurse.* Banbury: Lantern.

A mix of survival skills as a newly qualified nurse and as a new leader.

Jones, L and Bennett, CL (2012) *Leadership in Health and Social Care: An Introduction for Emerging Leaders.* Banbury: Lantern.

An easy to read general introduction to growing yourself as a leader.

Useful websites

www.businessballs.com/self-confidence-assertiveness.htm

A useful and interesting take on developing self-confidence.

http://changingminds.org/disciplines/change_management/psychology_change/ psychology_change.htm

A quirky but informative look at the psychology of change and transition.

http://changingminds.org/disciplines/change_management/kubler_ross/kubler_ross.htm

A useful introduction to the work of Kubler-Ross on the stages of grief during the dying process.

www.learnmanagement2.com/managementconcepts.htm

Some good pages on motivational theories can be found here.

www.mindtools.com/CommSkll/ActiveListening.htm

Some insights into active listening.

www.mindtools.com/pages/article/newTCS_82.htm

The Holmes and Rahe stress scale.

www.psychologytoday.com/basics/emotional-intelligence

A suite of very useful articles all about emotional intelligence.

Glossary

active listening   listening to, understanding and responding appropriately to what other people are saying.

binary thinking   in the sense used here it refers to a way of defining your identity with reference to the differences between you and someone else.

care pathways   detailed plans that map out what care a person with a particular need requires, as well as who will provide what at what stage.

charisma/charismatic   a facet of personality that is compelling to other people and inspires others to follow the individual who is charismatic.

clinical governance   the multiple methods of information gathering used to assess the quality of clinical care leading to improvements in the delivery and experience of care for the patient.

clinical supervision   a process of guided group reflection facilitated by a third party.

emotional intelligence   being aware of your own emotions, the emotions in others and how these modify behaviours, and being able to talk about this in a meaningful way with others.

Gantt chart   the most common format for displaying project outlines and progress. Named after Henry Gantt, who developed it in the early 1900s, the chart is a form of bar chart which displays activities or events plotted against time.

generalisability   the extent to which the findings of research apply to a wider population.

governance   the methods by which organisations follow regulations stipulated by higher governing bodies to ensure standards are met through their authoritative structures.

group think   a phenomenon that occurs when the members of a group make a collective decision based on seeking unanimity rather than encouraging individual reasoning or critical evaluation of ideas.

Hawthorne effect   changes that occur in people's behaviour because they know they are being observed.

Holmes–Rahe Life Event Rating Scale   a scale of 43 life events which are scored by the amount of stress they can cause. A high score means more stress. Some of the changes are positive ones but still cause significant stress.

integrity   staying true to your own moral and ethical principles.

learning cultures/organisations/teams   groups of people who learn from, and with, each other in the workplace, and use this learning to enhance what they do.

legitimate power   the power to lead and manage that an individual has by virtue of his or her position within an organisation, as well as the ability to use that power in a reasonable, perhaps ethical, manner.

mediation   resolution of conflict through the facilitation of an impartial third party.

negotiation/negotiate   the process of reaching a compromise agreement through talking.

operational   referring to the management of the day-to-day tasks of an organisation or team.

othering   the process whereby anyone who does not share the same characteristics as us is seen to be 'other'. If we are nurses, non-nurses are 'other'.

outcomes   in the sense they are used in this book, outcomes refer not only to the result of a care episode but also the individual's experience of care. Quality is therefore seen as achieving health goals as well as providing healthcare in a manner acceptable to and involving the client.

person-centred   referring to care that is provided with the needs and wants of the patients at its core. This is the opposite of providing care that is dictated by what health and social care professionals want to provide or which is rigidly dictated by policy.

quorate/quorum   the agreed number and designations of people needed to be at a meeting in order for it to make decisions, usually cited in the meeting's/committee's terms of reference.

skill mix   an appropriate number of people of various levels of ability on duty at the same time in order to be able to undertake the tasks required during a shift.

social capital   building up a bank of goodwill that can be called on later when you need a favour or support.

span of control   the number of employees for which each organisation manager or head of department is responsible.

stakeholders   individuals who will be affected directly or indirectly as a result of the organisation's actions, objectives, outcomes.

terms of reference   the purposes and powers of a committee, usually contained within a written document.

theory (pl. theories)   a logical attempt to explain a group of facts, phenomena or observations.

total quality management   an approach to quality management that takes account of both the outcome of the care episode and the ways in which the care episode was experienced by the patient or client.

values   the personal rules and understandings we have about what is right and what is wrong in human behaviour.

References

Abdelhafez, KH and Hossny, EK (2019) Nurses' perception of the first line nurse manager role as negotiator. *International Journal of Novel Research in Healthcare and Nursing*, 6(2): 1272–9.

Adair, J (1990) *How to Manage Your Time*. Guildford: Talbot Adair Press.

Adair, J (2010) *Develop Your Leadership Skills*. London: Kogan Page.

Antai-Otong, D (1997) Team building in a health care setting. *American Journal of Nursing*, 97 (7): 48–51.

Armstrong-Stassen, M, Freeman, M, Cameron, S and Rajacic, D (2015) Nurse managers' role in older nurses' intention to stay. *Journal of Health Organization and Management*, 29 (1): 55–74.

Attenborough, J, Abbott, S and Knight, R-A (2019) Everywhere and nowhere: Work-based learning in healthcare education. *Nurse Education in Practice*, 36: 132–8.

Barr, J and Dowding, L (2019) *Leadership in Healthcare*. London: Sage.

Barrick, MR and Mount, MK (1991) The big five personality dimensions and job performance: A meta analysis. *Personnel Psychology*, 44 (41): 1–26.

Bass, BM and Riggio, RE (2014) *Transformational Leadership: A Comprehensive Review of Theory and Research* (2nd edition). Hove: Routledge.

Bekirogullari, Z (2019) Employees' empowerment and engagement in attaining personal and organisational goals. *The European Journal of Social and Behavioural Sciences*, 26: 3032–47. https://doi.org/10.15405/ejsbs.264.

Belbin, MR (2010) *Management Teams: Why They Succeed or Fail* (3rd edition). Oxford: Butterworth Heinemann.

Benne, K and Sheats, P (1948) Functional roles of group members. *Journal of Social Issues*, 4: 41–9.

Benner, P (1984) *From Novice to Expert: Excellence and Power in Clinical Nursing Practice*. Menlo Park: Addison-Wesley.

Benner, P, Tanner, C and Chesla, C (2009) *Expertise in Nursing Practice: Caring, Clinical Judgment and Ethics* (2nd edition). New York: Springer.

Bennis, WG (1989) *On Becoming a Leader*. New York: Addison Wesley.

Bray, L and Nettleton, P (2007) Assessor or mentor? Role confusion in professional education. *Nurse Education Today*, 27 (8): 848–55.

Brennan, NM and Flynn, MA (2013) Differentiating clinical governance, clinical management and clinical practice. *Clinical Governance: An International Journal*, 18 (2): 114–31.

Brett, J and Thompson, L (2016) Negotiation. *Organizational Behavior and Human Decision Processes*, 136: 68–79.

Brewer, L (2019) *General Psychology: Required Reading*. Champaign: Noba.

Bridges, W and Bridges, S (2017) *Managing Transitions: Making the Most of Change* (4th edition). London: Nicholas Brearley.

Burnes, B (2017) *Managing Change* (7th edition). Oxford: Pearson Education.

Care Quality Commission (2020) *Cygnet Yew Trees Quality Report*. Available online at: www.cqc.org.uk/sites/default/files/new_reports/AAAK0090.pdf

Causer, G and Exworthy, M (2003) Professionals as managers across the public sector, in Bullman, A, Charlesworth, J, Henderson, J, Reynolds, J and Seden, J (eds) *The Managing Care Reader* (pp213–19). London: Routledge.

Chartered Institute of Personnel and Development (2020) *Performance Reviews Factsheet*. Available online at: www.cipd.co.uk/knowledge/fundamentals/people/performance/appraisals-factsheet

Chartered Institute of Personnel and Development (2021) *A Guide to Dealing with Conflict at Work*. London: CIPD.

Chicca, J and Shellenbarger, T (2018) Connecting with Generation Z: approaches in nursing education. *Teaching and Learning in Nursing*, 13(3): 180–4.

Chunta, KS (2020) New nurse leaders: creating a work-life balance and finding joy in work. *Journal of Radiology Nursing*, 39 (2): 86–8.

Clews, G (2010) *Lack of Support for Nurses Blamed for Mid Staffs Failings*. Available online at: www.nursingtimes.net/whats-new-in-nursing/acute-care/lack-of-support-for-nurses-blamed-for-mid-staffsfailings/5011861.article

Cornish, L and Holloway, S (2019) The role of the Healthcare Assistant in wound care. *Wounds UK*, 15 (5): 28–34.

Cummings, J (2012) *Leadership: What's in a Word?* Available online at: www.england.nhs.uk/tag/6cs

Curry, LA, Brault, MA, Linnander, EL, McNatt, Z, Brewster, AL, Cherlin, E, Flieger, SP, Ting, HH and Bradley, EH (2018) Influencing organisational culture to improve hospital performance in care of patients with acute myocardial infarction: a mixed-methods intervention study. *British Medical Journal: Quality and Safety*, 27: 207–17.

da Silva Copelli, FH, Erdmann, AL and Guedes los Santos, JL (2019) Entrepreneurship in nursing: an integrative literature review. *Revista Brasilera de. Enfermagem*, 72 (s1). https://doi.org/10.1590/0034-7167-2017-0523.

Daft, R (2001) *The Leadership Experience* (2nd edition). Florence, KY: South-Western Educational Publishing.

Darzi, A (2008) *High-Quality Care for All: NHS Next Stage Review Final Report.* London: Department of Health.

Davies, C (2004) Workers, professions and identity, in Henderson, J and Atkinson, D (eds) *Managing Care in Context* (pp189–210). London: Routledge.

Department of Health (1997) *The New NHS: Modern and Dependable.* London: DH.

Department of Health (2010) *Equity and Excellence: Liberating the NHS.* Available online at: www.gov.uk/government/uploads/system/uploads/attachment_data/file/213823/dh_117794.pdf

Dirks, KT and Ferrin, DL (2002) Trust in leadership: meta-analytic findings and implications for research and practice. *Journal of Applied Psychology,* 87 (4): 611–28.

Edwards, D, Burnard, P, Hannigan, B, Cooper, L, Adams, J, Juggessur, T, Fothergil, A and Coyle, D (2006) Clinical supervision and burnout: the influence of clinical supervision for community mental health nurses. *Journal of Clinical Nursing,* 15: 1007–10.

Ellis, P (2015) Delegating for success. *Wounds UK,* 11 (2): 70–1.

Ellis, P (2019a) *Understanding Research for Nursing Students (Transforming Nursing Practice)* (4th edition). London: SAGE.

Ellis, P (2019b) *Evidence Based Practice in Nursing (Transforming Nursing Practice)* (4th edition). London: SAGE.

Ellis, P (2020) *Understanding Ethics for Nursing Students (Transforming Nursing Practice)* (3rd edition). London: SAGE.

Ellis, P (2021a) Leadership approaches for modern nursing practice. *British Journal of Cardiac Nursing,* 16 (2): 1–5.

Ellis, P (2021b) How to manage difficult people (part 1): am I the problem? *Wounds UK,* 17 (1): 69–71.

Ellis, P and Abbott, J (2017) Developing yourself as a kidney care leader (part two). *Journal of Kidney Care,* 2 (5): 286–9.

Esterhuizen, P (2019) *Reflective Practice in Nursing (Transforming Nursing Practice)* (4th edition). London: SAGE.

Foster, S (2017) The benefits of values-based recruitment. *British Journal of Nursing,* 26 (10): 579.

Francis, R (2013) *Report of the Mid Staffordshire NHS Foundation Trust Public Inquiry.* Available online at: www.midstaffspublicinquiry.com/report

French, JPR Jr and Raven, B (1960) The bases of social power, in Cartwright, D and Zander, A (eds) *Group Dynamics* (pp607–23). New York: Harper and Row.

Gallwey, T (1974) *The Inner Game of Tennis.* New York: Random House.

Gallwey, T (2000) *The Inner Game of Work.* New York: Random House.

Garcia, AB, Rossi Rocha, FL, de Souza Cavalvante Pissinati, C, Palucci Marziale, MH, Henriques Camelo, SH and do Carmo Fernandez Lourenço Haddad, M (2017) The effects of organisational culture on nurses' perceptions of their work. *British Journal of Nursing*, 26(14): 806–12.

Gerardi, D (2015) Conflict engagement: workplace dynamics. *American Journal of Nursing*, 115 (4): 62–5.

Giddens, J (2018) Transformational leadership: what every nursing dean should know. *Journal of Professional Nursing*, 34 (2): 117–21.

Goleman, D (1996) *Emotional Intelligence: Why It Can Matter More Than IQ*. London: Bloomsbury.

Goleman, D (1998) *Working with Emotional Intelligence*. New York: Bantam Books.

Grant, A and Goodman, B (2018) *Communication and Interpersonal Skills in Nursing* (4th edition). London: SAGE.

Greer, LL, Van Bunderen, L and Yu, S (2017) The dysfunctions of power in teams: a review and emergent conflict perspective. *Research in Organizational Behavior*, 37: 103–24.

Griffin, RW (2016) *Management* (12th edition). Boston: Cengage Learning.

Griffiths, R (1983) *NHS Management Inquiry: Report to the Secretary of State of Social Services.* London: HMSO.

Grint, K (2020) Leadership, management and command in the time of the coronavirus. *Leadership*, 16 (3): 314–19.

Grint, K, Smolovic Jones, O and Holt, C. (2017) What is leadership: person, result, position, purpose or process or all or none of these? in Storey, J, Hartley, J, Denis, JL, Hart, P and Ulrich, D (eds) *The Routledge Companion to Leadership* (pp3–20). London: Routledge.

Handy, C (1994) *Understanding Organizations*. London: Penguin.

Handy, C (2020) *Gods of Management: The Four Cultures of Leadership*. Oxford: Oxford University Press.

Hardavella, G, Aamli-Gaagnat, A, Saad, N, Rousalova, I and Sreter, KB (2017) How to give and receive feedback effectively. *Breathe*, 13 (4): 327–33.

Harris, J and Mayo, P (2018) Taking a case study approach to assessing alternative leadership models in health care. *British Journal of Nursing*, 27 (11): 608–13.

Health and Safety Executive (nd) Health and Safety at Work etc. Act (1974). Available online at: www.hse.gov.uk/legislation/hswa.htm

Heeb, JL and Haberey-Knuessi, V (2014) Health professionals facing burnout: what do we know about nursing managers? *Nursing Research and Practice*. Available online at: doi:10.1155/2014/681814.

Her Majesty's Government (1998) Public Interest Disclosure Act. Available online at: www.legislation.gov.uk/ukpga/1998/23/contents

Her Majesty's Government (2005) Mental Capacity Act 2005. Available online at: www.legislation.gov.uk/ukpga/2005/9/contents

Her Majesty's Government (2008) Health and Social Care Act: Essential Standards of Quality and Safety. London: HMSO.

Her Majesty's Government (2010) Equality Act 2010. Available online at: www.legislation.gov.uk/ukpga/2010/15/contents

Her Majesty's Government (2018) *UK service economy: Blackett review.* Available online at: www.gov.uk/government/publications/uk-service-economy-blackett-review

Hersey, P, Blanchard, K and Johnson, D (2007) *Management of Organisational Behaviour* (9th edition). Oxford: Pearson Education.

Herzberg, F (1959) *The Motivation to Work.* New York: John Wiley.

Homans, GC (1961) *Social Behavior: Its Elementary Forms.* New York: Harcourt Brace.

Honey, P and Mumford, A (2006) *Learning Styles Questionnaire: 80-item Version.* London: Maidenhead.

Hopson, B and Adams, J (1976) *Transition: Understanding and Managing Personal Change.* London: Martin Robertson.

Interprofessional CPD and Lifelong Learning UK Working Group (2019) *Principles for continuing professional development and lifelong learning in health and social care.* Available online at: www.csp.org.uk/system/files/documents/2019-01/cpd_principles.pdf

Ion, R, Jones, A and Craven, R (2016) Raising concerns and reporting poor care in practice. *Nursing Standard,* 31(15): 55–62.

Jackson, C and Ellis, P (2010) Creative thinking for whole systems working, in Standing, M (ed) *Clinical Judgement and Decision Making in Nursing and Interprofessional Healthcare* (pp54–79). Maidenhead: Open University Press.

Janis, IL (1972) *Victims of Groupthink: A Psychological Study of Foreign-Policy Decisions and Fiascoes.* Boston: Houghton Mifflin.

Janis, IL (1982) *Groupthink: Psychological Studies of Policy Decisions and Fiascoes.* Boston: Houghton Mifflin.

Jug, R, Jiang, X and Bean, SM (2018) Giving and receiving effective feedback: a review article and how-to guide. *Archives of Pathology and Laboratory Medicine,* 143 (2): 244–50. doi: https://doi.org/10.5858/arpa.2018-0058-RA

Kelly, L, Lefton, C and Fischer, S (2019) Nurse leader burnout, satisfaction, and work-life balance. *The Journal of Nursing Administration,* 49 (9): 404–10.

Kim, S, Buttrick, E, Bohannon, I, Fehr, R, Frans, E and Shannon, SE (2016) Conflict narratives from the health care frontline: a conceptual model. *Conflict Resolution Quarterly,* 33: 255–77.

Kim, S, Bochatay, N, Relyea-Chew, A, Buttrick, E, Amdahl, C, Kim, L, Frans, L, Mossanen, M, Khandekar, A, Fehr, R and Lee, YM (2017) Individual, interpersonal, and organisational factors of healthcare conflict: a scoping review. *Journal of Interprofessional Care,* 31 (3): 282–90.

King's Fund (2015) *Leadership and Leadership Development in Health Care: The Evidence Base.* London: The King's Fund.

Kotter, J (1990) *A Force for Change: How Leadership Differs from Management.* New York: Free Press.

Kruse, K (2019) *Great Leaders Have No Rules.* New York: Rodale.

Lahana, E, Tsaras, K, Kalaitzidou, A, Galanis, P, Kaitelidou, D and Sarafis, P (2019) Conflicts management in public sector nursing. *International Journal of Healthcare Management,* 12 (1): 33–9.

Lewin, K (1951) *Field Theory in Social Sciences.* New York: Harper and Row.

Lingard, L, Sue-Chue-Lam, C, Tait, GR, Shad, J and Schulz, V (2017) Pulling together and pulling apart: influences of convergence and divergence on distributed healthcare teams. *Advances in Health Sciences Education,* 22: 1085–99.

Lorenz, EN (1963) Deterministic nonperiodic flow. *Journal of the Atmospheric Sciences,* 20 (2): 130–41.

Luft, J and Ingham, H (1955) The Johari Window, a graphic model of interpersonal awareness, in *Proceedings of the Western Training Laboratory in Group Development.* Los Angeles: UCLA.

Machell, S, Gough, P and Steward, K (2009) *From Ward to Board: Identifying Good Practice in the Business of the Caring.* London: King's Fund Publications.

Machell, S, Gough, P, Naylor, D, Nath, V, Steward, K and Williams, S (2010) *Putting Quality First in the Boardroom: Improving the Business of Caring.* London: The King's Fund and the Burdett Trust for Nursing. Available online at: www.kingsfund.org.uk/publications/putting-quality-first-boardroom

Magnusson, C, Allan, H, Horton, K, Johnson, M, Evans, K and Ball, E (2017) An analysis of delegation styles among newly qualified nurses. *Nursing Standard,* 31 (25): 46–53.

Manges, K, Scott-Cawiezell, J and Ward, MM (2017) Maximizing team performance: the critical role of the nurse leader. *Nursing Forum,* 52 (1): 21–9.

Manzano García, G and Ayala Calvo, JC (2021) The threat of COVID-19 and its influence on nursing staff burnout. *Journal of Advanced Nursing,* 77 (2): 832–44. https://doi.org/10.1111/jan.14642

Marquis, BL and Huston, CJ (2020) *Leadership Roles and Management Functions in Nursing: Theory and Applications* (10th edition). Philadelphia: Wolters Kluwer Health.

Maslach, C (2003) Job burnout: new directions in research and intervention. *Current Directions in Psychological Science,* 12 (5): 189–92.

Mayer, JD and Salovey, P (1993) The intelligence of emotional intelligence. *Intelligence,* 17 (4): 433–42.

McCloughen, A and Foster, K (2018) Nursing and pharmacy students' use of emotionally intelligent behaviours to manage challenging interpersonal situations with staff during clinical placement: a qualitative study. *Journal of Clinical Nursing,* 27 (13–14): 2699–709.

McKibben, L (2017) Conflict management: importance and implications. *British Journal of Nursing,* 26 (2): 100–03.

Merriman, C, Chalmers, L, Ewens, L, Fulford, B, Gray, R, Handa, R and Westcott, L (2020) Values-based interprofessional education: how interprofessional education and values-based practice interrelate and are vehicles for the benefit of patients and health and social care professionals. *Journal of Interprofessional Care*, 34 (4): 569–71.

Middleton, R, Moroney, T, Jackson, C and Germaine, R (2021) Education models embedding PD philosophy, values and impact: using the workplace as the main resource for learning, developing and improving, in Manley, K, Wilson, V and Øye, C (eds) *International Practice Development in Health and Social Care* (2nd edition; pp65–85). Hoboken: Wiley-Blackwell. https://doi.org/10.1002/9781119698463.ch6

Miller, L (2020) Remote supervision in primary care during the Covid-19 pandemic: the 'new normal'? *Education for Primary Care*, 31 (6): 332–6.

Mintzberg, H (1975) The manager's job: folklore and fact. *Harvard Business Review*, July/August: 66–75.

Morsiani, G, Bagnasco, A and Sasso, L (2017) How staff nurses perceive the impact of nurse managers' leadership style in terms of job satisfaction: a mixed method study. *Journal of Nursing Management*, 25 (2): 119–28.

Neergård, GB (2020) Entrepreneurial nurses in the literature: a systematic literature review. *Journal of Nursing Management*, 29 (5): 905–15. https://doi.org/10.1111/jonm.13210

Nelson-Brantley, HV and Ford, DJ (2017) Leading change: a concept analysis. *Journal of Advanced Nursing*, 73 (4): 834–46.

NHS Employers (n.d.a) *NHS Terms and Conditions (AfC) pay scales 2020/21*. Available online at: www.nhsemployers.org/pay-pensions-and-reward/agenda-for-change/pay-scales

NHS Employers (n.d.b) *Simplified Knowledge and Skills Framework (KSF)*. Available online at: www.nhsemployers.org/SimplifiedKSF

NHS England (2013) *Friends and Family Test*. Available online at: www.england.nhs.uk/ourwork/pe/fft/

NHS England (2014) *Five Year Forward View*. Available online at: www.england.nhs.uk/wp-content/uploads/2014/10/5yfv-web.pdf

NHS England and NHS Improvement (2019) *NHS Long Term Plan*. Available online at: www.longtermplan.nhs.uk/wp-content/uploads/2019/08/nhs-long-term-plan-version-1.2.pdf

NHS Improvement (nd) *About Us*. Available online at: https://improvement.nhs.uk/

NHS Improvement (2016) *Evidence from NHS Improvement on clinical staff shortages: A workforce analysis, February 2016*. Available online at: https://assets.publishing.service.gov.uk/government/uploads/system/uploads/attachment_data/file/500288/Clinical_workforce_report.pdf

NHS Leadership Academy (2013) *The Healthcare Leadership Model*. Available online at: www.leadershipacademy.nhs.uk/discover/leadershipmodel

NHS Survey Coordination Centre (2021) *NHS Staff Survey 2020.* Available online at: www. nhsstaffsurveys.com/Page/1056/Home/NHS-Staff-Survey-2020/

NMC (Nursing and Midwifery Council) (2017) *Revalidation.* Available online at: http:// revalidation.nmc.org.uk/welcome-to-revalidation

NMC (2018a) *Future Nurse: Standards of Proficiency for Registered Nurses.* Available online at: www.nmc.org.uk/globalassets/sitedocuments/education-standards/future-nurse-proficiencies.pdf

NMC (2018b) *The Code: Professional Standards of Practice and Behaviour for Nurses and Midwives.* London: NMC.

Nowell, L, White, D, Benzies, K and Rosenau, P (2017) Factors that impact implementation of mentorship programs in nursing academia: a sequential-explanatory mixed methods study. *Journal of Nursing Education and Practice,* 7 (10). https://doi.org/10.5430/jnep.v7n10p1

Nursing Standard (1985) Editorial: first nurses appointed DHA general managers. *Nursing Standard,* 385 (21 February): 1.

Olson, EE and Eoyang, GH (2001) *Facilitating Organization Change: Lessons from Complexity Science.* San Francisco: Jossey Bass/Pfeiffer.

Parry, E and Urwin, P (2017) The evidence base for generational differences: where do we go from here? *Work, Aging and Retirement,* 3 (2): 140–8. https://doi.org/10.1093/workar/waw037

Parsloe, E and Leedham, M (2009) *Coaching and Mentoring: Practical Conversations to Improve Learning.* London: Kogan Page.

Pascale, R (1990) *Managing on the Edge.* London: Penguin.

Patterson, C (2005) *Generational Diversity: Implications for Consultation and Teamwork.* Paper presented at the meeting of the Council of Directors of School Psychology Programs on generational differences. Deerfield Beach, Florida.

Perlman, AI and Abu Dabrh, AM (2020) Health and wellness coaching in serving the needs of today's patients: a primer for healthcare professionals. *Global Advances in Health and Medicine.* doi:10.1177/2164956120959274

Qalehsari, MQ, Khaghanizadeh, M and Ebadi, A (2017) Lifelong learning strategies in nursing: a systematic review. *Electron Physician,* 9 (10): 5541–50.

Raghubir, A (2018) Emotional intelligence in professional nursing practice: a concept review using Rodgers's evolutionary analysis approach. *International Journal of Nursing Sciences,* 5 (2): 126–30.

Redshaw, G (2008) Improving the performance appraisal system for nurses. *Nursing Times,* 104 (18): 30–1. Available online at: www.nursingtimes.net/nursing-practice-clinical-research/improving-theperformance-appraisal-system-for-nurses/1314790.article

Robinson-Walker, C (2020) *Leading with Mastery and Heart: The Coaching Companion for Thriving Nurse Leaders.* London: Elsevier.

Ross, L and Meier, N (2021) Improving adult coping with social isolation during COVID-19 in the community through nurse-led patient-centered telehealth teaching and listening interventions. *Nursing Forum,* 1–7. https://doi.org/10.1111/nuf.12552

Salmela, S, Koskinen, C and Eriksson, K (2017) Nurse leaders as managers of ethically sustainable caring cultures. *Journal of Advanced Nursing*, 73 (4): 871–82.

Salvage, J and White, J (2019) Nursing leadership and health policy: everybody's business. *International Nursing Review*, 66 (2): 147–50.

Sanko, J, McKay, M, Shekhter, I, Motola, I and Birnbach, DJ (2020) What participants learn, with, from and about each other during inter-professional education encounters: a qualitative analysis. *Nurse Education Today*, 88: 104386. https://doi.org/10.1016/j.nedt.2020.104386

Scammell, J (2018) Do you take your breaks? How to influence change in the workplace. *British Journal of Nursing*, 27 (9): 514. doi: 10.12968/bjon.2018.27.9.514

Scaria, MK (2016) Role of care pathways in interprofessional teamwork. *Nursing Standard*, 30 (52): 42–7.

Scholtes, PR (1998) *The Leader's Handbook: A Guide to Inspiring Your People and Managing the Daily Workflow*. New York: McGraw-Hill.

Schuetze, H and Inman, P (2010) *The Community Engagement and Service Mission of Universities*. Leicester: National Institute of Adult and Continuing Education (NIACE).

Schwartz, SH (1994) Are there universal aspects in the structure and contents of human values? *Journal of Social Issues*, 50 (4): 19–45.

Senge, P (1990) *The Fifth Discipline: The Art and Practice of the Learning Organization*. New York: Doubleday.

Senge, P (1996) Leading learning organizations. *Training and Development*, 50 (12): 36–7.

Setyaningrum, RP, Setiawan, M, Fueb, S and Irawanto, DW (2020) Servant leadership characteristics, organisational commitment, followers' trust, employees' performance outcomes: a literature review. *European Research Studies Journal*, 23 (4): 902–11.

Smola, KW and Sutton, CD (2002) Generational differences in working age women. *Journal of Organizational Behavior*, 23 (4): 363–82.

Snowdon, DA, Leggat, SG and Taylor, NF (2017) Does clinical supervision of healthcare professionals improve effectiveness of care and patient experience? A systematic review. *BMC Health Service Research*, 17: 786. https://doi.org/10.1186/s12913-017-2739-5

Storkholm, MH, Mazzocato, P and Savage, C (2019) Make it complicated: a qualitative study utilizing a complexity framework to explain improvement in health care. *BMC Health Services Research*, 19: 1. https://doi.org/10.1186/s12913-019-4705-x

Sullivan, EJ and Decker, PJ (2009) *Effective Leadership and Management in Nursing* (7th edition). Harlow: Pearson International Edition.

Tamunomiebi, M and Uhuru, G (2018) Group, teams and tasks in the organization: a historical escortion. *European Journal of Business and Management Research*, 3 (4). Available online at: doi: 10.24018/ejbmr.2018.3.4.15

Thomas, KW and Kilmann, RH (1974) *Thomas–Kilmann Conflict Mode Instrument*. Sterling Forest, NY: Xicom.

Tian, X and Yue Wang, T (2014) Tolerance for failure and corporate innovation. *The Review of Financial Studies*, 27 (1): 211–55. https://doi.org/10.1093/rfs/hhr130.

Tuckman, BW (1965) Developmental sequence in small groups. *Psychological Bulletin*, 63: 384–99.

Tuomikoski, AM, Ruotsalainen, H, Mikkonen, K and Kääriäinen, M (2020) Nurses' experiences of their competence at mentoring nursing students during clinical practice: a systematic review of qualitative studies. *Nurse Education Today*, 85: 104258. https://doi.org/10.1016/j.nedt.2019.104258

van Breda-Verduijn, H and Heijboer, M (2016) Learning culture, continuous learning, organizational learning anthropologist. *Industrial and Commercial Training*, 48 (3): 123–8. https://doi.org/10.1108/ICT-11-2015-0074.

von Bertalanffy, L (1968) *General System Theory: Foundations, Developments, Applications.* New York: Braziller.

Welch-Horan, TB, Lemke, DS, Bastero, P, Leong-Kee, S, Khattab, M, Eggers, J, Penn, C, Dangre, A and Doughty, CB (2021) Feedback, reflection and team learning for COVID-19: development of a novel clinical event debriefing tool. *BMJ Simulation and Technology Enhanced Learning*, 7 (1): 54–7.

Whitmore, J (1992) *Coaching for Performance: GROWing Human Potential and Purpose: The Principles and Practice of Coaching and Leadership. People skills for professionals.* Boston: Nicholas Brealey.

Wright, P (1996) *Managerial Leadership.* London: Routledge.

Yoder-Wise, P (2019) *Leading and Managing in Nursing* (7th edition). Maryland: Mosby.

Index

Locators in *italics* refer to figures and those in **bold** to tables.

3 D technique 115–116
6 Cs 40
360-degree appraisal 139, **140**

accommodating (conflict management) 101
accountability 20, 61, 72
action-centred leadership 40–42, *41*
active listening 102–103, 179
Adair's action-centred leadership 40–42, *41*
Agenda for Change (AfC) 75, 141
Antai-Otong, D. 61
anxiety 62, 95, 148
appraisals 78–81, 138–141, **140**
    see also performance management
arbitration (conflict management) 104

Belbin, Meredith 56–57
Big five personality theory 81-82
binary thinking 95–97
Blanchard, K. 112, 113
board level nurses 134–135
Bray, L. 118
Brennan, N. M. 137
bullying 97–99
burnout 124

care pathways 66
care quality *see* quality of care
Care Quality Commission (CQC) 135–137
centralisation (organisational structures) 133–134
challenging situations 184–185
    see also conflict management
change management 141–142
    complexity and chaos theory 146–148
    entrepreneurship 148–150
    PDSA model 145
    steps of change 144–145
    theory of 143–144
chaos theory 147
charisma 15, 19–20
Chartered Institute of Personnel and Development
    (CIPD) 97, 138
clinical governance 135–137
clinical supervision
    appraisals **140**
    conflict management 93
    definition 119–120
    learning culture 111

coaching
    3 D technique 115–116
    appraisals **140**
    GROW technique 115
    to improve performance 111–115
    learning culture 111
    and mentoring 117
The Code 21, 35, 72
collaboration (conflict management) 101
committees 63–65
communication
    environments of care 156
    self-management 106
    within the team 62
    understanding ourselves 14
    understanding situations 179–180
competency *see Future Nurse: Standards of Proficiency for*
    Registered Nurses
competing (conflict management) 101
complexity theory 146–148
compromising (conflict management) 101
conflict management
    arbitration 104
    binary thinking 95–97
    confronting challenging
        situations 184–185
    importance of 92–94
    managing situations 100–102
    managing yourself 105–106
    meaning of 91–92
    mediation 103
    negotiation 102–103
    reducing the potential for
        conflict 99–100
    sources of conflict 90, 94–99
    teamwork 53, 61
    whistle blowing 104–105
contingency theory 32
COVID-19
    burnout 124
    change management 142, 146
    clinical supervision 120
    leadership 15, 16
    policy context 21
    and values 13
cultural diversity 83
culture *see* learning environments; organisational
    culture

Darzi report 134
decentralisation (organisational structures) 133–134
delegation 73–75, 112–113
dodging (conflict management) 101

emotional intelligence
    conflict management 100
    leadership 185
    role of 44–45
    self-management 106
entrepreneurship 148–150
environments of care 155–157
Equity and Excellence: Liberating the NHS 135
ethics
    generational differences 85–86
    workload management 35–36
    see also values
extroversion 82

feedback
    appraisals 79–81
    patient experience 135
    teamwork 53–54, 57, 61
flexible working 125
Flynn, M. A. 137
Francis report 105, 134
Future Nurse: Standards of Proficiency for Registered Nurses 3
    assessing needs and planning care 89–90, 110,
        129–130
    being an accountable professional 4, 25, 69, 89, 109,
        129, 153, 170
    coordinating care 5, 49
    leading and managing nursing care and working in
        teams 5, 25–26, 49, 70, 110, 153–154, 170–171
    providing and evaluating care 69–70, 130
    role models 183
    safety and quality of care 70, 130, 149, 171

Gallwey, Tim 114
Gantt charts 144–145
generational differences 84–86
goals
    change management 144–145
    GROW technique 115
    management by objectives **140**
    quality of care 134, 136–137
    self-motivation 177
Goleman's emotional intelligence framework 44–45
governance 135–137
group think 64–65
GROW technique 115

harassment 93, 99
Hardavella, G. 80–81
Hawthorne effect 33
health and safety 93, 105
healthcare assistants (HCAs) 75–76, 80
Healthcare Leadership Model 43–44
Hersey, P. 112, 113
hierarchical structures 133–134
Holmes-Rahe Life Event Rating Scale 176
Homans, George 57, *58*

individual performance 71
    appraisals 78–81, 138–141, **140**
    feedback 53–54
    individual roles, responsibility and accountability
        72–73
    pay bands 141
    personal development plans 77–78
integrity 16–17
    see also values
intelligence 15
    see also emotional intelligence
interdisciplinary teams 65–67
intrapreneurism 149

job satisfaction 177–179
Johari window 13–14, *14*, 86

Knowledge and Skills Framework 75, 141
Kotter, J. 76, 112

leadership
    characteristics of a good leader 15–17
    confidence 172, 178–179
    context and values 6–11
    delegation 73–75, 76–77
    developing yourself 177–185
    distinction from management 26–29
    in health and social care 26
    Healthcare Leadership Model 43–44
    how we see ourselves and others see us 13–15
    individual, cultural and generational differences
        81–86
    as a nurse 1–2, 17–20
    policy context 20–21
    professional-management continuum 172–173
    skill mix 75–76
    within teams 72
    theories of 37–43
    transitions 172–176
    values 5–11, 15–17, 182–183
    what happens when values are forgotten? 11–13
leadership style 112
learning environments 154–155
    clinical supervision 111
    developing a learning environment 164–168
    elements of 161–164
    importance of 158–161
    leadership 157
    lifelong learning 117, 119, 156–158, 166
    meaning of 157–158
    values 123, 168
learning organisations 100, 121–123
legitimate power 17–18, 19–20
Lewin, Kurt 143
lifelong learning 117, 119, 156–158, 166
listening skills 102–103, 179

management
    characteristics of a good manager 15–17
    distinction from leadership 26–29
    in health and social care 26
    policy context 20–21

resilience 36–37
theories of 29–34
values and assumptions 5–6
workload management 34–36
Manchester Clinical Supervision Scale (MCSS) 124
Maslach Burnout Inventory (MBI) 124
mediation (conflict management) 103
meetings 63–65
mentoring
in healthcare 117
learning culture 111
multiprofessional views 118
outside of healthcare 118–119
mentors 117, 119
Mintzberg's management role theory 30–32
mistake-making 180–181
moral practice 35–36
see also values
motivation
Hawthorne effect 33
motivation-hygiene theory of job satisfaction
177–179
self-motivation 177
transformational leadership 39–40
motivation-hygiene theory of job satisfaction 177–179

National Institute for Health and Care Excellence
(NICE) 21
National Vocational Qualifications (NVQs) 75
Neergård, G. B. 149
negotiation (conflict management) 102–103
Nettleton, P. 118
NHS Improvement 137–138
NHS Leadership Model 43
NMC guidance 21
norms
generational differences 84–86
organisational culture 82–83
teamwork 55
nursing
board level nurses 134–135
leadership 1–2, 17–20
professionalisation of 154
nutrition 80

organisational culture 82–83
conflict management 100
learning and development 158
NHS Leadership Model 43
and values 12–13
see also learning environments
organisational governance 135–137
organisational structures 131–134
othering 95–97

patient experience 135
Patterson, C. 84, 85–86
pay bands 141
PDSA model 145
peer review 139, **140**

perceptions
how we see ourselves and others see us 13–15
teamwork 62
values and assumptions about leadership 5–6
performance management 71
appraisals 78–81, 138–141, **140**
feedback 53–54
individual roles, responsibility and accountability
72–73
pay bands 141
personal development plans 77–78
performance review 138
personal development plans 77–78
personality traits 62, 81–82
PEST analyses 30
PESTLE analyses 30
policy context 20–21
power
conflict management 95
legitimate power 17–18, 19–20
management role theory 30
meetings and committees 63
organisational culture 158
practice assessors 117
practice supervisors 117, 159–160
professional development
leadership development 177–185
leadership transitions 172–176
learning organisations 121–123
lifelong learning 119, 156–158
skill mix 121–122
via delegation 76–77
professional standards *see Future Nurse: Standards of
Proficiency for Registered Nurses*
professionalisation of nursing 154
psychiatric case management 66–67
Public Information Disclosures Act 105
*Putting Quality First in the Boardroom: Improving the
Business of Caring* report 135

Qualifications and Credit Framework (QCF) 75
quality of care
as goal 134, 136–137
NHS Improvement 137–138

recruitment 59, 92, 161
refreezing (change management) 143–144, 145
relationships
appraisals 80
building up 53, 58–60
see also teamwork
resilience 36, 183–184
responsibility, lines of 17–19
rewards (performance management) 141
role models 40, 117, 157, 183
roles (teams) 55–57, **56**
rosters 35, 104

Scaria, M. K. 66
self-appraisal 79

self-assessment (appraisals) 139, **140**
self-awareness 13–15, 43, 114, 185
self-belief 180
self-development 160, 177–185
    see also professional development
self-management 105–106, 126
self-motivation 177
servant leadership 42–43
situational leadership model 112, 114
skill mix 75–76, 121–122
social exchange theory 58
social systems, influence on teamwork 57–58, *58*
span of control 132
staff development *see* professional development
stakeholders 143
standards *see Future Nurse: Standards of Proficiency for Registered Nurses;* quality of care
stress
    burnout 124
    resilience 36, 183–184
    teamwork 62
    work-life balance 126
student nurses
    group norms 55
    leadership transitions 172–176
    learning environments 163
    self-awareness 185
    understanding context 7–8
    values 11
supportive teams 45–46
systems theory 32–34, 57

teamwork
    communication within the team 62
    group think 64–65
    how teams work 50–52
    individual, cultural and generational differences 81–86
    influence of social systems 57–58, *58*
    interdisciplinarity 65–67
    leadership role 72
    managing problems 61
    meetings and committees 63–65
    NMC Standards of Proficiency 49
    supportive teams 45–46
    team dynamics and processes 54–57
    team effectiveness 52–54, **54**, 58–60
    workload management 35
time management 34–36, 123–124, 181–182
total quality management 93
trainee nurses *see* student nurses
trait-rating scales **140**
transactional leadership 38
transformational leadership 38–40
transitions 172–176
trust 38–40, 45–46
    confidence as a leader 178–179
    conflict management 99–100
    good leaders 45–46
    transformational leadership 38–39
    values 182
Tuckman, B. W. 51

unfreezing (change management) 143, 144

values
    and assumptions 5–6
    and context 6–11
    definition 9
    how we see ourselves and others see us 13–14
    integrity 16–17
    leadership and management 5–6, 15–17, 182–183
    learning environments 123, 168
    what happens when values are forgotten? 11–13
vulnerability 95

waiting times 91–92, 93–94
From Ward to Board report 135
whistle blowing 104–105
work-based learning 158–159
work-life balance 125–126
workload management 34–36, 123–124, 181–182